ADVANCE PRAISE FOR
Food Allergies: A Complete Guide for Eating When Your Life Depends on It

"An indispensable book for anyone who has food allergies or any parent of a child with food allergies. As an allergist treating food-allergic patients every day, I keep this book within easy reach on my bookshelf. It's a unique source of knowledge for those of us who treat such patients."

PHIL LIEBERMAN, M.D.
Clinical Professor of Medicine and Pediatrics
Division of Allergy and Immunology
University of Tennessee College of Medicine

"A must-read for teens and adults with food allergies, and for anyone living with or caring for someone with food allergies. Here they will find answers to many of their questions as well as interesting case histories and essential principles of diagnosis and treatment, including a realistic overview of future approaches."

F. ESTELLE R. SIMONS, M.D.
University of Manitoba
Past-President, American Academy of Allergy, Asthma & Immunology
Past-President, Canadian Society of Allergy, Asthma & Immunology
Chair, World Allergy Organization Special Committee on Anaphylaxis

"Dr. Sicherer draws on his years of experience as a master clinician, researcher, author, and thought leader in this field to provide practical advice and countless insights that are sure to provide the reader with the knowledge needed to understand and manage food allergies. The question-and-answer format makes this comprehensive book highly accessible to people with food allergies and parents of children with food allergies, while the extensive insights and depth of detail make it an important resource for health care providers as well. Dr. Sicherer describes in detail how to integrate food allergies into a family lifestyle. A family's ability to anticipate a food reaction and then treat the symptoms if they happen—and not expect a reaction to happen all the time—helps a family cope thoughtfully with food allergies in a child."

A. WESLEY BURKS, M.D.
Chair of Pediatrics, University of North Carolina
President, American Academy of Allergy, Asthma & Immunology

"In this definitive guide to food allergies, Scott Sicherer offers his readers a complete food allergy education. He demystifies everything from science to symptoms to label reading and offers encouragement for living life to its fullest—in spite of food allergies. Destined to be the go-to resource for patients and parents striving to live well with food allergies."

GWEN SMITH
Editor, *Allergic Living* magazine

"Dr. Sicherer answers all the questions parents and others have about food allergies. From practical considerations to emotional issues to the latest in the search for a cure—it's all here. The easy-to-read question-and-answer format will make this a reference book you reach for time and again. I wholeheartedly recommend it!"

ANNE MUÑOZ-FURLONG
Founder, The Food Allergy & Anaphylaxis Network
(now Food Allergy Research & Education)

"*Food Allergies: A Complete Guide for Eating When Your Life Depends on It* is required reading for patients, parents, and physicians who want to help patients who have food allergies—young or old. Parents should keep a copy of this book next to *Understanding and Managing Your Child's Food Allergies* (also by Dr. Sicherer) so they can better understand food allergies, obtain better medical care, and ultimately enjoy a better quality of life. As a parent of children with life-threatening food allergies, these are my essential reference books."

AMIE RAPPOPORT MCKENNA
Mother of children with severe food allergies

FOOD ALLERGIES

A Johns Hopkins Press Health Book

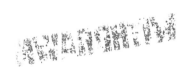

FOOD ALLERGIES

A COMPLETE GUIDE FOR EATING WHEN YOUR LIFE DEPENDS ON IT

SCOTT H. SICHERER, M.D.

Foreword by Maria Laura Acebal, Food Allergy Research & Education (formerly The Food Allergy & Anaphylaxis Network)

Introduction by Hugh A. Sampson, M.D., Jaffe Food Allergy Institute, Mount Sinai School of Medicine

THE JOHNS HOPKINS UNIVERSITY PRESS

BALTIMORE

Medical disclaimer. This book is not meant to substitute for medical care of people with allergies, and treatment should not be based solely on its contents. Instead, treatment must be developed in a dialogue between the individual and his or her physician. This book has been written to help with that dialogue. The author and publisher are not responsible for any adverse consequences resulting from the use of information in this book.

Drug dosage. The author and publisher have made reasonable efforts to determine that selection and dosage of drugs discussed in this text conform to the practices of the general medical community. The medications described do not necessarily have specific approval by the U.S. Food and Drug Administration for use in the diseases and dosages for which they are recommended. In view of ongoing research, changes in governmental regulations, and the constant flow of information relating to drug therapy and drug reactions, the reader is urged to check the package insert of each drug for any change in indications and dosage and for warnings and precautions. This is particularly important when the recommended agent is a new and/or infrequently used drug.

Copyright © 2013 Scott H. Sicherer, M.D.
All rights reserved. Published 2013 by the Johns Hopkins University Press
Printed in the United States of America on acid-free paper
9 8 7 6 5 4 3 2 1

The Johns Hopkins University Press
2715 North Charles Street
Baltimore, Maryland 21218-4363
www.press.jhu.edu

Library of Congress Cataloging-in-Publication Data

Sicherer, Scott H.
   Food allergies : a complete guide for eating when your life depends on it / Scott H. Sicherer ; foreword by Maria Laura Acebal ; introduction by Hugh A. Sampson.
      p. cm.
   Includes bibliographical references and index.
   ISBN 978-1-4214-0844-6 (hdbk. : alk. paper) — ISBN 978-1-4214-0845-3 (pbk. : alk. paper) — ISBN 978-1-4214-0898-9 (electronic) — ISBN 1-4214-0844-9 (hdbk. : alk. paper) — ISBN 1-4214-0845-7 (pbk. : alk. paper) — ISBN 1-4214-0898-8 (electronic)
   1. Food allergy—Diet therapy. I. Title.
   RC588.D53S56 2013
   616.97'30654—dc23   2012025274

A catalog record for this book is available from the British Library.

The Food Allergy Action Plan is reprinted with permission from Food Allergy Research & Education (formerly the Food Allergy & Anaphylaxis Network); www.foodallergy.org.

Special discounts are available for bulk purchases of this book. For more information, please contact Special Sales at 410-516-6936 or specialsales@press.jhu.edu.

The Johns Hopkins University Press uses environmentally friendly book materials, including recycled text paper that is composed of at least 30 percent post-consumer waste, whenever possible.

CONTENTS

xi Foreword, by Maria Laura Acebal

xiii Preface

xv Introduction, by Hugh A. Sampson, M.D.

Chapter 1.   1
What Are the BASIC FACTS about Food Allergy?

1 Allergy and Other Adverse Reactions to Foods

3 Symptoms and Illnesses

8 Severity

9 When Symptoms Are Not a Food Allergy

10 Masqueraders of Food Allergy

14 Prevalence of Food Allergies

15 Causes and Triggers of Food Allergies

17 Peanuts

18 Eggs

20 Cow's Milk

24 Wheat and Other Grains

25 Tree Nuts

29 Seeds

30 Soy

32 Legumes

33 Vegetables and Starches

34 Fruits

35 Meats

36 Fish

38 Shellfish

40 Spices

41 Alcoholic Beverages

42 Miscellaneous Food Allergens and Colors, Additives, and Preservatives

46 When to Seek Help

47 Delving Deeper: Latex and Food Allergies

47 Also of Interest: Unusual Food Reactions

Chapter 2.   49
What Do I Need to Tell the Doctor to
Help Get a FOOD ALLERGY DIAGNOSIS?

49 When to Talk to Your Doctor

50 How to Prepare for a Doctor Visit

54 Finding the Right Doctor and Other Health Professionals

56 Delving Deeper: Alternative Therapies

58 Also of Interest: Tests to Avoid

Chapter 3.   59
These Food ALLERGY TESTS Are Confusing!
What Do They Mean?

59 General Questions about Testing

60 Skin Tests

67 Blood Tests (and How They Compare with Skin Tests)

74 Elimination Diets

77 Oral Food Challenges (Feeding Tests)

84 Additional Tests

86 Unproven and Disproven Tests

88 Delving Deeper: Improved Diagnostic Tests and Component Testing

90 Also of Interest: Reasons for Unexpected Test Results

Chapter 4.   91
What Is ANAPHYLAXIS and How Do I Treat It?

91 General Questions on Anaphylaxis

101 Epinephrine

108 Antihistamines

111 Additional Medications and Treatments for Anaphylaxis

113 Written Emergency Plans, Education, Medical Identification Jewelry,
     Management Issues

115 Delving Deeper: Predicting Anaphylaxis and Taking a Treatment Quiz

118 Also of Interest: Exercise and Anaphylaxis

118 Answers to Delving Deeper: Anaphylaxis Treatment Quiz

Chapter 5. 120
What CHRONIC HEALTH PROBLEMS Are Caused by Food Allergy?

120 General Questions about Chronic Illnesses and Foods

121 Respiratory Symptoms

121 Hives

124 Atopic Dermatitis (Eczema)

127 Gastrointestinal, Digestive Illnesses

128 Colic, Constipation, Irritable Bowel Syndrome, and Reflux

132 Celiac Disease (Gluten-Sensitive Enteropathy)

133 Proctocolitis (Food Protein–Induced Proctocolitis)

135 Food Protein–Induced Enterocolitis Syndrome

141 Food Protein Enteropathy and Protein Intolerance

141 Eosinophilic Esophagitis and Other Eosinophilic Gut Diseases

147 Delving Deeper: Delayed Allergic Reactions

147 Also of Interest: Chronic Illnesses That Are Not Related
     to Food Allergies

Chapter 6. 149
How Do I AVOID ALLERGIC REACTIONS to Foods?

149 General Questions about Avoiding Allergic Reactions

151 Cross-Contact

152 Amounts That Trigger a Reaction and Casual Exposure

157 Avoidance at Home

159 Purchasing Manufactured Products

164 Restaurants

168 Social Outings and Family Gatherings

169 School

184 Camp

185 Work

186 Travel

188 Dating and Relationships

189 Age-Related Responsibilities

192 Special Exposure Risks

195 Delving Deeper: Risks and Risk Reduction Controversies

195 Also of Interest: The Peanut-Sniffing Dog

Chapter 7.   197
How Do I Manage a Food Allergy While Living a Normal and Healthy LIFESTYLE, with ADEQUATE NUTRITION?

197 General Questions on Lifestyle and Quality of Life

199 Emotional Concerns and Anxiety

204 Interpersonal Relationships and Bullying

207 Nutrition

213 Delving Deeper: An Allergic Reaction's Effect on Quality of Life

213 Also of Interest: Anxiety Reactions

Chapter 8.   214
Will These Food Allergies Ever GO AWAY?

214 General Questions about Food Allergy Resolution

215 The Course of Allergies to Specific Foods

217 The Course of Illnesses Caused by Food Allergies

218 Evaluations for Resolution of Food Allergy

219 Recurrence of a Food Allergy and Development of New Food Allergies

220 Factors Affecting the Course of Food Allergies

221 Delving Deeper: Resolution of Food Allergies

222 Also of Interest: The Air-Food Connection

Chapter 9.   223
Is There Any Way to PREVENT Food Allergies?

223 General Questions on Prevention

228 Pregnancy Diets

229 Breast Feeding and Formulas

232 Introducing Solid Foods

233 Current Recommendations

235 Nondietary Aspects of Prevention

237 Delving Deeper: Difficulties in Studying Allergy Prevention

238 Also of Interest: Insights on Prevention from Worldwide Observations

Chapter 10.
Will There Be a CURE or BETTER TREATMENT of Food Allergy?

239 General Questions about Food Allergy Research

243 Approaches to Treat Any Type of Food Allergy

246 Approaches to Treat Allergies to Specific Foods

251 Treatments of Specific Food-Allergic Diseases

251 Unproven Treatments

254 Participating in Food Allergy Research

258 Delving Deeper: Chinese Herbal Therapies

259 Also of Interest: Why Has Research Been So Slow?

Chapter 11.
How Do I Get MORE HELP and INFORMATION to Manage Food Allergies?

260 Educational Resources

266 Support Groups, Advocacy, and Research

267 Handy Forms

270 Selected Medical References

273 Index

FOREWORD

Maria Laura Acebal

Former CEO, The Food Allergy & Anaphylaxis Network

Our family's introduction to food allergies began with a tiny bite of an orange-colored peanut butter cracker and ended with a rush to the emergency room, where not just one but two doses of epinephrine were required to stop our toddler's anaphylactic reaction. I'd had no idea a food allergy could be so serious; after that day, I had no doubt.

Like the millions of families that receive this life-changing diagnosis, we had so many questions. Where to begin? And even now, with more than eight years of living with food allergies under our belt —and my work at the Food Allergy & Anaphylaxis Network—we still encounter new doubts, new milestones, new challenges that shake our sense of comfort and leave us searching for clear guidance.

This book provides that guidance and more. I found answers to important questions I hadn't yet thought of asking. From practical advice on school safety, traveling, eating out, and dating, to the scientific underpinnings of the search for a cure and the emotional toll of food allergies on families, the topics covered are the ones that most affect our lives. No matter what part of this journey you are on—whether you received the diagnosis only hours ago or have been living with food allergies for years—you will learn so much by reading this book.

And you couldn't be learning it from a better source. Dr. Sicherer is one of the world's most respected voices on food allergies. He is not only a leading clinician but also a respected researcher, who has dedicated his career to making life better and safer for all those living with food allergies.

Long before meeting Dr. Sicherer and having the honor and pleasure of working with him professionally, I knew him as the author of *Understanding and Managing Your Child's Food Allergies*, one of my most relied-on books. As a new food allergy mom, I turned to this earlier work time and again, gaining so much confidence from his good counsel. Now, in this new book, he delivers his ever-growing expertise in a most accessible, easy-to-read format that puts the explanations and practical information you need right at your fingertips.

Destined to be earmarked and underlined, these pages are an incredible resource for food-allergic individuals as well as for parents, families, and schools—in short, anyone who cares about someone with food allergies. And, because I love someone with food allergies, I will recommend it for years to come.

PREFACE

This book is dedicated to people with food allergies and those who care for them. It is the result of thousands of questions I have been asked by adults and children with food allergies, parents of children with food allergies as well as allergists, medical students, physicians in training, pediatricians, the media, government officials, researchers, teachers, school nurses, and others. Your questions have led me at times to seek answers from you as well as from others, from research, and through trial-and-error experiences. It is my pleasure and privilege to present this book designed to give you what you have asked for: a place to find accurate, timely, detailed, and helpful answers to questions on every aspect of food allergies.

Of course, this book would not exist were it not for the work and influences of many people, and so I also dedicate this volume to the many who have taught me over the years, including Hugh A. Sampson, M.D., Anne Muñoz-Furlong, Sally Noone, R.N., Marion Groetch, R.D., Robert A. Wood, M.D. (whom I also thank for his critical review of the manuscript), my many colleagues at Mount Sinai's Jaffe Food Allergy Institute, and researchers and colleagues worldwide. I want to thank the Food Allergy Initiative, for proving that a group of concerned parents can address the need for more research and awareness with resounding success, and the Food Allergy & Anaphylaxis Network, for bringing educational materials to those who need them; these two groups have since merged to become Food Allergy Education & Research. Thanks to the Jaffe family, for their foresight in establishing a food allergy institute at Mount Sinai in New York, and to the National Institute of Allergy and Infectious Diseases, for funding the Consortium of Food Allergy Research. I thank my wife, Mati, and children, Andrew, Zachary, Maya, Sydnee, and Cassaddee . . . for everything.

INTRODUCTION

Hugh A. Sampson, M.D.
Director, Jaffe Food Allergy Institute, Mount Sinai School of Medicine,
New York, New York

Over the past 31 years, I have been fortunate to witness and participate in a remarkable evolution in our understanding of food allergies. When I began my food allergy research in the early 1980s, I approached the disorder by applying my background in detailed scientific methods. Although a bit reluctant and highly skeptical, I was encouraged to explore this area by Dr. Susan Dees, an emeritus professor and a wonderful mentor during my early years at Duke University. Then my own fascination with the field grew due to experiences with my second daughter, who had food allergies, eczema, and later asthma, and as I cared for an increasing number of families and children with food allergy symptoms in my clinical practice. In those early years, I was reluctant to admit to my colleagues that I was focusing my research on food allergy. The reason for my trepidation was that food allergy, in those early days, was considered not a "real disease" but a problem of little consequence. Part of the reason for this misperception was that many people were attributing various problems to foods that were never proven to be involved using scientifically validated methods. At the same time, people were not recognizing allergic diseases that actually were caused or worsened by foods. Although everyone acknowledged that a food could cause a severe allergic reaction, the life-threatening nature of this allergy was not well appreciated.

In the mid-1970s, the food allergy field began to emerge from scientific uncertainty in part because of the work of Drs. Charles May and Allan Bock, who emphasized the need to use a diagnostic procedure called a *double-blind, placebo-controlled oral food challenge*, which is discussed in detail in this book. This test brought objectivity to the diagnosis of food allergies by eliminating patients' and physicians' preconceived notions. In my research work, the procedure fostered incredible scientific advances to further improve the diagnosis and treatment of food allergies. Food allergy became "real" and was now viewed as a medical illness worthy of attention and acknowledged as a field of allergy in need of more research. Today food allergy has become a hot topic, and many programs around the world are actively pursuing a better understanding of these disorders and effective forms of therapy.

The emergence of food allergy from the "dark ages" into a time of scientific exploration was exciting; however, the past two decades have unfortunately witnessed an alarming increase in food allergies and other allergic diseases. For reasons we do not fully understand, allergic diseases have become much more common, particularly in westernized societies. Our studies estimate that over 11 million Americans now have food allergies, and about 5 million of these are children. Children are experiencing more food allergies that persist longer than when I began to study this disease. The burden of living with food allergies remains largely untold and underappreciated. Those who are allergic and their families must practice constant dietary caution and be at the ready to treat severe allergic reactions. Despite increasing awareness, this disease is still sometimes fatal.

Although the increase in food-allergic disease has been disheartening, the challenges posed have been met with increasing efforts to improve life for those affected. Twenty years ago, Anne Muñoz-Furlong established the Food Allergy & Anaphylaxis Network (FAAN), which has become a tremendous resource on every aspect of living with food allergies. FAAN's numerous triumphs have resonated throughout government agencies, legislation, industry, and various health care organizations to raise awareness and improve life for those with food allergies. FAAN has become a model for similar groups globally. The Food Allergy Initiative in New York and the Jaffe Food Allergy Institute established the precedent that parents and the public can affect the research enterprise. By raising funds to support food allergy research, they have stimulated national funding agencies to follow suit and increase research spending in this important area. Remarkable advances have been made, understanding has increased, and the future is looking brighter. But a piece has still been missing.

The increase in people suffering with food allergies along with the explosion of information (and misinformation) about food allergy has outpaced our ability to teach food allergy sufferers, parents, children, and caregivers what we have learned. Being unable to find reliable information with sufficient details about food allergies leaves patients, parents, and other caregivers feeling unfulfilled and confused. They have many burning questions and concerns. We now have clear answers for many of these concerns, and when the right answer is unclear, we have plenty of information that can be helpful while research is under way. Knowing the answers and understanding the issues behind what we can't answer yet are vital to working with your doctor, discussing your or your child's food allergy with others, and ultimately obtaining the best care possible. This book is an amazing compilation of the essential information you need to do this, and it is the only resource I know of that provides timely, accurate, and accessible information on every medical aspect of food allergy.

Dr. Scott Sicherer has culled nearly two decades of experience in patient care and research to present this information in a readable and easily understandable format. He provides both basic medical information and tips on how to deal with everyday issues such as visiting the allergist, dealing with schools and restaurants, navigating the supermarket, and so forth. As an internationally recognized leader in food allergy education and research, Dr. Sicherer has been at the cutting edge of clinical and social issues of food allergy. As a lecturer, he has had countless discussions about food allergy experiences with patients, parents, school nurses, camp directors, food service professionals, pediatricians, internists, allergists, children, and many others. He has distilled these experiences here to answer virtually every possible question about food allergies, from questions you may have wondered about to, more important, many questions you should be asking.

The information in this book is so comprehensive and timely that it should be required reading not only for adults with food allergies and parents of children with food allergies, but also for physicians, teachers, school nurses, camp personnel, spouses, and everyone who plays a role in caring for those with food allergies. It will help them to understand and more effectively and safely manage these allergies, which is why I certainly plan to keep a copy in my clinic and to recommend it to the many people I encounter whose lives are affected in some way by these pervasive allergies to food.

FOOD ALLERGIES

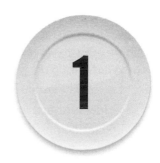

What Are the

BASIC FACTS

about Food Allergy?

This chapter answers questions about what a food allergy is and how to recognize symptoms. I explain how food allergies differ from other illnesses caused by foods. I describe various types of food allergies and the foods that cause them. Many of the concepts introduced in this chapter are discussed in more detail in subsequent chapters.

ALLERGY AND OTHER ADVERSE REACTIONS TO FOODS

What is a food allergy?
A food allergy happens when the immune system attacks harmless proteins in foods.

What is the immune system?
The immune system is the part of the body that normally fights germs. It is composed of various cells and proteins.

How does the immune system "attack" proteins in foods?
Two ways: with cells that release various chemicals or by producing proteins, called IgE antibodies.

What role do the IgE antibodies play in food allergy?

The most common forms of food allergy, when allergic reactions happen suddenly after a food is eaten, are the result of the immune system making IgE antibodies. These proteins are like small antennae that sit atop allergy cells (called mast cells and basophils) and detect the food proteins. The IgE "antennae" are able to detect a specific food protein, for example a peanut protein or an egg protein. When these IgE antibodies come in contact with the food protein, they signal the allergy cells to release powerful chemicals, such as histamine, which produce allergic symptoms.

How do cells in the immune system cause food allergies?

The cells respond to the food protein by releasing chemicals that cause inflammation with persistent symptoms, such as rashes, or symptoms affecting the gut, such as pain, nausea, and vomiting. The term "non-IgE–mediated," or "cell-mediated," food allergy is used when the cells of the immune system are causing allergic responses to foods without involving IgE.

Other than food allergy, how might foods make a person sick?

A food can make a person ill in many ways. Food poisoning happens when bacteria in spoiled food releases toxins that can cause symptoms. Chemicals in foods can cause symptoms in some people. For example, caffeine may cause sweating, tremors, or heart palpitations. Food intolerance causes some people to become ill from a food that does not trouble others.

What is a food intolerance?

Unlike a food allergy, intolerance does not involve the immune system. It is a problem that affects people who have trouble digesting certain sugars in foods. For example, beans have a sugar that is difficult to digest. This is why beans are "gassy" foods. Lactose intolerance, a problem digesting milk sugar, is the most common. It is caused by a deficiency of lactase enzyme, which digests lactose sugar.

At what age does a person develop a food allergy?

Any age. However, food allergies most often develop in infancy and childhood.

What are the most common triggers of food allergy in infants, children, and adults?

For infants and children, cow's milk, eggs, and peanuts are the most common triggers, followed by tree nuts, shellfish, soy, wheat, and fish. Adult-onset food allergy usually involves nuts, seafood, fruits, or vegetables.

How do I know if I have a food allergy?

Specific symptoms after eating a food, or patterns of symptoms, are a good clue that you may have a food allergy.

SYMPTOMS AND ILLNESSES

What symptoms should make me suspect a food allergy?

Having sudden allergic symptoms within an hour or two of eating a food should raise suspicions of a food allergy. However, allergic reactions can also be more insidious. A food allergy can cause chronic daily symptoms that may be more difficult to connect to particular foods.

What are common sudden symptoms of a food allergy?

Sudden allergic symptoms (also called *acute symptoms*) can affect the skin with rashes such as hives (like mosquito bites), swelling (especially of the face and lips), itching, and flaring of eczema rashes. Symptoms can affect breathing with throat tightness, repetitive coughing, wheezing, swelling of the throat and tongue, difficulty swallowing, and trouble getting air in and out. The gut can be affected with pain, nausea, vomiting, and diarrhea. There may be itchiness in the mouth and throat, or an odd taste such as a metallic one. Women may feel uterine contractions. When blood circulation is impaired, the heart may beat very fast or very slow, skin may turn pale or blue, the pulse may be difficult to feel, blood pressure may be low, and there can be confusion, dizziness, light-headedness, and passing out. Sometimes in a severe allergic reaction, a person has a feeling of impending doom.

What are common chronic symptoms of a food allergy?

When foods cause a constant inflammation in the body, the person may have chronic rashes of allergic eczema, also called atopic dermatitis. There may be gut symptoms of vomiting, pain, or diarrhea; poor growth in children; or weight loss in adults.

What types of medical illnesses are caused by food allergy?

Several medical illnesses result from sudden or chronic food-allergic reactions. These go by many different medical terms, including anaphylaxis, oral allergy syndrome, eczema, proctocolitis, enterocolitis, enteropathy, eosinophilic esophagitis, contact hives, occupational food allergy, food-associated exercise-induced anaphylaxis (FAEIA), and others. I devote entire chapters in this book to considering the details of many of these problems.

What is anaphylaxis?

Anaphylaxis is a severe allergic reaction that is rapid in onset and can be fatal. Typically, several areas of the body are affected, for example, the skin and the gut, or the gut and breathing. Chapter 4 is devoted to questions about anaphylaxis.

What is oral allergy syndrome / pollen-associated food allergy syndrome?

A person with this type of allergy is initially allergic to proteins in pollens and then has symptoms when eating certain raw fruits or vegetables that have similar proteins in them (not on them). A pollen-allergic person would not normally clean a pollen-covered car by licking it, but if he did his tongue might get very itchy. Biting into an apple that is rich with pollen-like proteins can lead to the same uncomfortable mouth symptoms. The problem occurs only with raw forms of fruits and vegetables because heating the food destroys the problematic proteins.

What are examples of the pollen and food relationships in oral allergy syndrome?

Birch pollen proteins are related to rock fruits, those with pits, including apples, pears, peaches, plums, and cherries, as well as to vegetables such as carrots and celery. Ragweed pollen proteins are related to melons and bananas. Mugwort is related to spices such as fennel, celery, coriander, and parsley. Many people with pollen allergies have no symptoms, and those who do have symptoms vary greatly from each other in which foods bother them.

Can oral allergy syndrome be severe?
Rarely. About 1% or 2% experience more severe reactions, and about 7% have symptoms beyond the mouth. One reason reactions are usually mild is that people generally stop eating the food if it bothers them too much.

Can a person with oral allergy syndrome eat the food anyway?
Many people with oral allergy syndrome eat the raw foods if they are not too uncomfortable. Additionally, the heated forms (applesauce, peach pie, canned fruits, cooked carrots, etc.) should be tolerated.

How can food be rendered less likely to trigger a reaction in oral allergy syndrome?
The easiest means is to heat the food. Some people get relief from briefly microwaving the food, peeling the fruit, or dipping the fruit in lemon juice.

Is there seasonal variation in oral allergy syndrome?
The symptoms tend to increase during the relevant pollen season and fade or improve after. Therefore, when your eyes and nose are itchiest in the pollen season, you are more apt to have problems eating the related raw fruits or vegetables. When you are at the longest period away from your pollen season—just before the season begins the following year—the symptoms from eating the problem foods should be at their minimum.

Why do some foods bother a person with oral allergy syndrome and other related ones do not?
It is remarkable that people with the same pollen allergy can have symptoms with different related foods or with none at all. We do not know the reason for this variation.

*Can a person with oral allergy symptoms from one type of apple
tolerate different types?*

Surprisingly, yes. For example, a person may have no symptoms from Fuji apples but become quite itchy from Granny
Smith. This is probably because different types of apples vary in the
amounts of the relevant proteins as well as in the degree of similarity to
the pollens. Additionally, the allergenic proteins tend to increase with
longer storage times, so fresher apples may be less of a problem.

How do doctors treat oral allergy syndrome?

Allergists differ in whether they have their patients avoid these foods,
with many making case-by-case decisions based on the person's history of
reactions. For example, the more discomfort someone has felt, the more
likely a doctor will advise the person to avoid the food. Taking antihistamines might reduce symptoms. Some studies suggest that immunotherapy (allergy shots) against the related pollens may also reduce symptoms.

Are symptoms of oral allergy to nuts more concerning?

Nuts are in general more likely than fruits and vegetables to cause severe
allergic reactions. However, some nuts have pollen-related proteins and
fall into the same category as other pollen-related food allergens, perhaps
indicating less risk of a severe reaction. Almonds, hazelnuts, and peanuts
have pollen-related proteins, so they may cause relatively mild allergies
for some people. Since these foods are known to trigger severe reactions,
however, an allergist may suggest that a person who's had any symptoms
should avoid them entirely. Studies are under way to improve diagnostic
tests to differentiate which proteins, the mild or more problematic, a person is more reactive to in these foods. Until then, decisions are likely to be
individualized, with your allergist considering your past reactions, other
allergies, and personal preferences.

What is food-related atopic dermatitis, or eczema?

Atopic dermatitis, or allergic eczema, is a chronic skin condition in which
the skin is dry, rashy, and very itchy. About one in three children with
worse than mild forms of the rash also have food allergies.

What are proctocolitis, enterocolitis, and enteropathy?

These are gut allergies that usually begin in infancy and have symptoms such as vomiting, diarrhea (sometimes bloody), pain, and poor growth, depending on the particular illness. Most people outgrow these types of allergies during childhood. Cow's milk is the most common trigger.

What are eosinophilic esophagitis and eosinophilic gut disease?

Eosinophilic gut disease results from a chronic allergic inflammation in the lining of the digestive tract. Swelling and breakdown of the gut lining result in symptoms, which vary depending on what area of the gut has swelling. For example, inflammation in the esophagus (eosinophilic esophagitis), the tube connecting the mouth to the stomach, causes pain when food is swallowed, and food may get stuck in the tube. For most people with this illness, food is the main trigger of the inflammation.

What are contact hives?

When a food touches the skin directly and results in hives where the food made contact, these are called contact hives, also known as contact urticaria. This term is usually reserved for situations when a food, although tolerated when eaten, causes symptoms only on skin contact. Contact urticaria occurs most often in infants and young children, when messy eating results in hives around the mouth but the food is otherwise tolerated. Common triggers are acidic fruits, such as tomatoes and strawberries.

What is food-associated exercise-induced anaphylaxis?

People with this problem can exercise without any allergic symptoms. They can also eat without symptoms. But if they eat foods, or a particular food, and then exercise, they develop allergic symptoms and possibly anaphylaxis. Common triggers are wheat, celery, and shellfish.

What are occupational food allergies?

These allergies are related to exposure on the job, usually to large amounts of food, and often through the skin or air. Baker's asthma describes a situation where wheat flour in the air triggers wheezing, although the baker can eat wheat products. People working with fruits or vegetables might develop skin rashes from the exposure, with the rashes flaring from skin contact with the food. Many different foods can cause occupation-related reactions.

SEVERITY

How severe can a food allergy be?
Food allergies can be fatal.

Do allergic reactions worsen each time a food is eaten?
No. This is a common misconception. Subsequent reactions could be more severe, less severe, or equal in severity.

Is severity of a food allergy predictable?
No, although there are some patterns. Certain foods are more likely to cause dangerous reactions. For example, peanut, tree nut, shellfish, and fish allergies are usually more severe than fruit or vegetable allergies. Severity may be related to the amount eaten, with more dangerous symptoms following a larger amount ingested. Having co-existing asthma is also a risk factor for more extreme reactions.

Why is having asthma a risk factor for more severe reactions?
Asthma is linked to more severe reactions most likely because the lung is more vulnerable to wheezing symptoms during a food-allergic reaction.

How many people die from food allergies?
We do not have exact numbers, but it appears to be uncommon. Some researchers have calculated that more people die from lightning strikes. However, fatalities do occur, most often striking teenagers and young adults. It is important to realize that these tragedies are preventable. Avoiding severe and fatal allergic reactions to foods requires education about avoidance, and knowing how and when to treat an allergic reaction.

WHEN SYMPTOMS ARE NOT A FOOD ALLERGY

What common medical problems do people wrongly attribute to food allergy?
Various maladies have been attributed to food allergies despite the link being unproved or even being disproved. Symptoms and illnesses with which a relationship to food allergy remains controversial or unproven include behavioral and developmental problems in children, headaches, and weight gain. Some illnesses that are attributed to food "allergy" may actually be triggered by the chemical components of the foods, not really an allergy. Additionally, allergic symptoms are sometimes wrongly attributed to foods when a different allergic cause is the culprit.

What are examples of allergic conditions that can be wrongly attributed to a food allergy?
Food and nonfood triggers of allergic symptoms can cause the same symptoms, which can lead to confusion. For example, hives can be triggered by a virus. Wheezing and nasal symptoms of itching, sneezing, and congestion are often triggered by allergens in the air, such as pollens or animal dander. Chronic rashes can be triggered by irritants such as soaps, infections, sweating, or allergens in the air.

Can foods affect behavior?
Possibly, but not typically through allergy. Caffeine in foods may cause irritability or increased activity because of a pharmacologic (drug) effect. Sugar does not appear to affect behavior. Some studies support the notion that chemical colors and preservatives adversely affect some children's attention or trigger hyperactivity, but this is not attributed to allergy. Rather, the connection is purported to be caused by the chemical effects of these additives. If a true food allergy affected behavior, it would likely do so only indirectly, such as through chronic disruptive symptoms, like itchy rashes, that interrupt sleep.

Can foods cause headaches?
Possibly, but not through allergy. Chemicals in some foods, such as fer-

mented foods and hard cheeses, may trigger migraines in some people, but this is not an allergic reaction.

Can a food allergy cause weight gain?

This is a common misconception, especially attributed to wheat. Severe allergies are more likely to cause weight loss or poor weight gain, because the gut does not respond properly. Cakes and cookies may result in weight gain, but this is because of their calories, not an allergy!

Can food allergy cause fatigue?

Not specifically. However, a person with chronic malnutrition and allergic symptoms due to food allergies may become fatigued from the illnesses.

MASQUERADERS OF FOOD ALLERGY

I have trouble breathing, develop tingling and numbness in my fingers, and feel light-headed. Is this a food allergy?

This group of symptoms certainly shares some features with an allergic reaction. However, these are also common symptoms of breathing quickly and deeply, a problem called hyperventilation.

How does hyperventilation mimic a food allergy?

When a person hyperventilates, such as from anxiety, changes in the chemicals in the bloodstream can cause symptoms. The light-headedness, trouble breathing, and general discomfort are similar to symptoms of a food-allergic reaction. Calming down and breathing into a bag should help. This situation can mimic a food-allergic reaction especially if a person is concerned about possible exposure to an allergenic food, which leads to anxiety and possible hyperventilation.

I notice blistering and burning on my skin in the summer when I have gin and tonic. Is that an allergy?

The sun and the lime juice, not an allergy, are causing the blistering and burning. There are chemicals in limes, lemons, celery, parsnip, and parsley that are called psoralens. When these are on the skin and exposed to the sun, a chemical reaction may occur that results in a burn, with blistering and redness over the next few days. This may occur on the hands of people preparing the drinks or foods or on the lips of those eating or drinking the foods. To avoid this reaction, wash off the juices right away and avoid the sun when working with or ingesting foods with psoralens in them.

My nose runs after eating hot or spicy foods. Is that an allergy?

The chemical that makes some foods hot or spicy can also trigger a runny nose through a neurologic response. Some people are more sensitive to this than others. Sometimes the temperature of a food, for example, steaming hot beverages or soups, will trigger runny nose symptoms, again based on neurologic, not allergic, responses.

I often sneeze while eating breakfast, no matter what the food. Is this an allergy?

There are many triggers of sneezing in the morning. A buildup of mucus from the night before can trigger a sneeze. Another cause of morning sneezing is sunlight. As the sun flickers through the window, it can trigger a neurologic response in some people that makes them sneeze.

When I ate fish, I had allergic symptoms, but so did others at the table. Is that an allergy?

This description fits scombroid fish poisoning. When dark-meat fish like tuna or mahi mahi spoils, it can develop histamine-like toxins. Histamine is the chemical made by allergy cells that cause allergic symptoms. When the histamine-like toxin from the spoiled fish is eaten, a person may experience symptoms of mouth and throat itching, stomach pain, and skin redness that fully mimic an allergic reaction.

My child develops a red streak on her face when she eats certain foods. Is that an allergy?

If there is no swelling or itching, and the red streak always develops in the same area, it may be something called auriculotemporal syndrome, also known as Frey syndrome or gustatory flushing. This is a neurologic response resulting from minor nerve damage. Rarely, this happens on both sides. The streak runs from the corner of the mouth to the ear on one side of the face when a food promotes salivation. Tart or sour foods are the most likely triggers. The nerve damage results in a connection between salivation and the nerves that tell blood vessels in the cheek to expand, causing more redness.

Children at risk are those born by forceps delivery, presumably having experienced some nerve trauma to the face. This usually fades with age. Adults with this problem are usually those treated for salivary gland cancer, with resulting nerve damage.

I notice gas, bloating, and loose stools when I have dairy. Is this a milk allergy?
No, it is more likely to be lactose intolerance.

What is lactose intolerance?
A difficulty in digesting the sugar, called lactose, in milk, because of a deficiency in an enzyme called lactase, is called lactose intolerance. Without sufficient lactase enzyme, the lactose passes along the intestine undigested and unabsorbed. Gut bacteria can get a hold of the lactose and ferment it, causing gas. The extra sugar in the intestine can draw fluids out of the body and into the gut, causing diarrhea.

Who is at risk for lactose intolerance?
After infancy and early childhood, most of us gradually lose our ability to digest lactose. Having a lactase deficiency in adulthood is actually a normal situation, although the degree varies among different races and ethnicities. Persons of Asian descent have the highest rates of lactase deficiency, over 90%. Of Native Americans and African Americans, over 70% have lactase deficiency. The lowest rates, 5% to 20%, are among Caucasian adults. The rate at which lactase levels decrease over time as a person ages is also racially and ethnically related. For example, within a few years after breast feeding, Chinese and Japanese lose 80% to 90%, while Jews

and Asians lose 60% to 70%. White Northern Europeans may reach their lowest level of lactase after age 20. Having a stomach virus can also result in temporary loss of lactase for days or weeks.

What foods cause symptoms of lactose intolerance?
Any food with milk. Dairy products normally contain about 4% to 5% lactose by weight, enough to create symptoms in lactose intolerant people. However, different foods may have different amounts. Cheese and yogurt often do not lead to symptoms because lactic acid bacteria in the foods help to digest the lactose. Some cheeses contain less lactose, including camembert, cheddar, cream cheese, and parmesan.

How much milk sugar causes symptoms when a person has lactose intolerance?
This is very variable, with some people being sensitive to tiny amounts and others being able to have many ounces before symptoms appear.

How is lactose intolerance diagnosed?
Usually through trial and error, seeing if reducing lactose in the diet relieves symptoms. However, a medical diagnosis can be confirmed with testing, using a breath hydrogen test performed by drinking lactose and having a breath test to check for poor absorption.

How is lactose intolerance treated?
By reducing the lactose. This is accomplished either by dietary reduction or avoidance, purchasing lactose-free milk products, or using replacement enzymes that are available over-the-counter.

What other foods cause this type of intolerance?
Beans contain a sugar that is hard to digest, giving them a reputation for causing gas. That is why enzymes are sold to reduce gas from eating beans. Some people have trouble absorbing a sugar called fructose, especially in foods with lower amounts of glucose, another sugar. The symptoms can include gas, diarrhea, and abdominal pain. Problem foods include apples, pears, fruit juices, watermelon, raisins, honey, foods with high fructose

corn syrup, wheat-containing foods, sorbitol, artichokes, leeks, and on-ions. A doctor can diagnose this problem using a breath hydrogen test.

PREVALENCE OF FOOD ALLERGIES

How common are food allergies?

More than 1% but less than 10% of the population is estimated to have food allergies, with 4% to 8% of children and 3% to 4% of adults affected. If the estimate includes very mild food allergies, the total percentage of people affected may be closer to 10%.

Is there really an increase in food allergies, or is there just more awareness or publicity?

No one knows for sure. Several studies support the conclusions of most experts that there truly has been an increase over the past few decades. Studies that I have been involved in suggest a tripling in peanut allergy among children between 1997 and 2008, now with more than 1 in 100 children affected.

Why does one person develop a food allergy and another does not?

Genetic predisposition (allergies run in families) and environmental fac-tors (exposure to foods, components of the diet, and other factors) play a role.

Why would the body attack foods if it only results in damage and bad reactions?

I agree that no obvious good comes from having food allergies. One theory is that the attack on foods is a misdirected one. The part of the immune system that is activated against proteins in foods is the same part that fights parasite, or worm, infections. Perhaps persons who develop aller-gies would be well protected if they lived in a setting with parasites, but otherwise, their immune systems' responses to harmless proteins, such as those in foods, are counterproductive.

CAUSES AND TRIGGERS OF FOOD ALLERGIES

What foods cause food allergies?
Any food. Over 170 have been noted to cause a reaction.

What are the most common foods to trigger allergies?
Milk, eggs, peanuts, tree nuts, shellfish, fish, wheat, and soy account for the most significant allergies. Allergies to fruits and vegetables are usually less severe. Allergies to seeds, such as sesame, are being increasingly reported.

Aren't strawberries, tomatoes, chocolate, and corn common food allergens?
These foods have been frequently listed as common allergens, but they are far from the most common true allergic triggers. People may experience problems with these foods because some of them have chemicals with irritant properties that cause mild allergy-like symptoms. These reactions are often inconsistent, and a person may have mild symptoms only sometimes when eating the food.

Do children have different food allergy triggers than adults?
Yes. Children are more likely to have allergies to milk, egg, wheat, and soy. These are not common allergens in adults, partly because they are usually outgrown during childhood. Infants and young children are not likely to have developed allergies related to raw fruits and vegetables because these are pollen-related allergies (see oral allergy syndrome discussed earlier), and people typically have to experience a few pollen seasons to become allergic.

Can a person be allergic to fats?
No. However, a person may have trouble digesting fats.

Can a person be allergic to sugars?
No. People are not allergic to simple sugars in foods.

Can a person be allergic to iodide?

No. There is a misconception that an "iodide" allergy is at the root of both seafood allergies and allergies to injected dyes used for radiographic medical tests. However, iodide does not trigger typical allergic reactions such as hives, wheezing, or anaphylaxis. In fact, iodide is in salt, which we all eat.

Why do we hear so much about peanut allergy?

Peanut allergy is widespread and usually persistent, and it accounts for most of the reported fatal reactions to foods. Additionally, peanuts are a common ingredient in foods and therefore difficult to avoid.

If I am allergic to one food, does that mean I will be allergic to related foods?

The answer depends on the food group. For example, peanuts are a type of legume, or bean, but 95% of people with a peanut allergy can eat other types of beans. On the other hand, a person with an allergy to one type of crustacean shellfish, such as shrimp, has a more than 50% chance of being allergic to other types, such as lobster and crab.

If a food is organic or farm raised, does that change the allergic potential?

No. The proteins are the same.

Does cooking a food make it less allergenic?

The answer depends on the food. Some foods appear to become more likely to trigger an allergic reaction (increased allergenicity) when heated. For example, roasting peanuts appears to make the proteins more capable of triggering an allergic response. In contrast, heating fruits and vegetables usually makes them less allergenic for people with protein-induced food allergies. How the proteins in foods behave when heated can also vary by how the food is heated, the temperature, and the associated ingredients. For example, frying peanuts does not appear to make them as allergenic as roasting. Boiling milk does not appear to significantly change its allergenic properties, but heating it in the airy environment of a cake may alter some of the proteins, reducing their allergenicity.

What do I need to know about allergies to specific foods?

When you know you have an allergy to a food, you need to know whether to worry about related foods. Understanding some features of certain foods can help you better understand potential risk of allergy and how to avoid reactions. The questions and answers that follow address major food allergens, common food groups, and food additives.

PEANUTS

What kind of food are peanuts?

They are beans (legumes).

If I have a peanut allergy, do I need to avoid all beans?

Usually not, because 95% of people with a peanut allergy tolerate other beans, such as soybeans, peas, string beans, and so on.

Are any foods more risky for people with a peanut allergy?

Children with a peanut allergy are at increased risk of having other food allergies, but not necessarily to nuts or beans, with one exception. Lupine, a type of bean, appears more likely to be allergenic for people with a peanut allergy (about a 20% risk).

What is lupine?

Lupine, also called lupin, can be found in many gluten-free, high-protein, and specialty food products, such as pastas and breads. In parts of Europe and Australia, lupine flour is often mixed with wheat flour in baked goods.

What foods might have peanuts in them?

Peanuts are ubiquitous. They may be found in many manufactured products, such as candy, chocolate, baked goods, and ice creams. Ethnic restaurants (such as Chinese, African, Indonesian, Thai, and Vietnamese), bakeries, and ice cream parlors use peanut in many foods. Peanut butter or peanut flour may be used as a "secret" ingredient to thicken and flavor chili and spaghetti sauce.

Are peanuts used in nonfood items?
Yes, peanuts may be found in, for example, cosmetics, nutritional supplements, medicines, and pet foods.

Is peanut oil safe for a person with peanut allergy?
It may be, but I usually advise against routinely using peanut oil. Peanut protein is found in unrefined peanut oils that are cold pressed, expressed, expelled, and extruded from peanut. These oils are unsafe. Highly refined peanut oils contain only the fat left over after the protein is removed. These oils should be safe, but it may be difficult to identify the type of oil used in a product. Therefore, I usually recommend avoidance of peanut oil or extreme care in making sure the safe peanut oil is used.

Can a person with a peanut allergy eat tree nuts?
No significant proteins are similar between peanut and tree nuts. Although most people with a peanut allergy will tolerate some or all tree nuts, many tree nuts (such as pecans, walnuts, almonds, etc.) are processed with peanuts and therefore may contain trace amounts of peanut protein, making these foods risky. Candies and chocolates also are often processed with peanuts. Therefore, for practical purposes, many individuals and families choose to avoid tree nuts and most candy and chocolate when there is a peanut allergy. Options for eating tree nuts despite having a peanut allergy are discussed further in chapter 6.

EGGS

Are people allergic to the egg white or yolk?
The proteins most likely to cause allergic reactions are found in the white. However, most allergists suggest avoiding both the white and the yolk because it is difficult to separate these components in cooking.

If I am allergic to chicken eggs, do I need to avoid other types of eggs?
Yes. People with chicken egg allergy are likely to be allergic to other poultry eggs, like quail.

Does having a chicken egg allergy mean that I would be allergic to fish eggs?
No.

Can people with an egg allergy eat foods that have eggs baked into them, such as muffins or waffles?
About 70% of people with an egg allergy can tolerate small amounts of egg in baked goods like cookies.

Why can some people with an egg allergy eat eggs in baked forms?
The process of heating the egg in an "airy" environment alters the proteins. For some people, this is enough to make the food safe to eat. This is different than simply baking an egg. There may also be a difference in the amount of egg being consumed, with baked goods having less.

If I am allergic to eggs and have not tried to eat eggs in baked goods, can I try these foods?
NO. You need to discuss this with your allergist. A severe reaction is possible (unless you are already eating those products successfully).

What words or ingredients might indicate that a food contains eggs?
U.S. labeling laws require use of the word "egg" on product ingredient labels. Words that may refer to eggs as ingredients are albumin, lysozyme (used in Europe), egg (white, yolk, dried, lecithin, powdered, solids), mayonnaise, meringue, eggnog, ovalbumin, ovovitellin, and globulin.

What foods might have eggs in them?
Eggs may be found in baked goods, breaded foods, cream fillings, custards, candies, canned soups, casseroles, eggnog, frostings, ice creams, lollipops, marshmallows, marzipan, nougat, pastas, salad dressings, and meat-based dishes such as meatballs or meatloaf. Egg whites and shells may be used as clarifying agents in soup stocks, consommés, bouillons, wine, and coffees. A shiny glaze on baked goods may be an "egg wash."

Can I use an egg replacer or egg substitute if I have an egg allergy?
Be careful! Don't get tricked. Most "egg substitutes" contain eggs.

Are eggs used in nonfood items?
Yes. Eggs may be found in cosmetics, nutritional supplements, medicines, and pet foods.

What vaccines have egg in them?
There is not enough egg in the measles, mumps, and rubella vaccine (MMR) to cause an allergic reaction. Therefore, this vaccine poses no greater risk to people with an egg allergy than it does to people without one. The yearly influenza vaccine has trace egg protein, but most people can get the immunization anyway, so ask your doctor. People traveling to areas where contracting yellow fever is a risk might need a vaccine that contains egg. A person with an egg allergy would need to be given this vaccine only under special circumstances by an allergist.

What medications have egg in them?
An anesthetic agent called propofol has a fatty derivative from eggs; the medical literature is unclear on whether this is a risk, but so far it appears unlikely. Otherwise, egg is not a common ingredient in medications, but it is prudent to check any medication for inclusion of food allergens.

COW'S MILK

What proteins in milk cause milk allergies?
Milk contains many proteins, including casein and whey. The casein proteins appear to be the most potent allergens, but often a person with a milk allergy reacts to many of the proteins in milk. Even if whey proteins are tolerated, most foods with milk in them, including those listing only whey ingredients, have some amount of casein in them as well.

If I have a cow's milk allergy, can I drink other types of mammalian milks, like goat's milk?
If you are allergic to cow's milk, then you are almost certainly (>90%) allergic to milk from goats, sheep, and other mammals. Equine milks (donkey, mare) are less like cow's milk and allergenic to only about 10% of people with a cow's milk allergy, but these milks are not widely available.

Are other foods a concern for a person with a milk allergy?
Among people with severe cow's milk allergy, about 10% may react to beef, especially if it is rare because some proteins that cause allergy in some people are in both the cow's milk and blood.

Can people with a milk allergy eat foods that have milk baked into them, such as muffins, or can they tolerate some cheeses?
About 70% of people with milk allergy can tolerate smaller amounts of milk in baked goods like cookies. Some people can even tolerate some cheese (which is heated but not baked).

Why can some people with a milk allergy eat milk in baked forms?
The process of heating the milk in an "airy" environment alters the proteins. For some people, this is enough to make the food safe to eat. These effects don't occur when simply heating a glass of milk.

If I am allergic to milk and have not tried to eat milk in baked goods, or cheese, can I try these foods?
NO. You need to discuss this with your allergist. A severe reaction is possible (unless you are already eating those products successfully).

What terms might indicate that a food contains milk, or is a dairy food?
U.S. labeling laws require that the term "milk" be used if it is an ingredient. Milk shows up in all sorts of foods, so watch out for artificial butter flavor, butter fat, butter oil, butter, casein and caseinates (in all forms), cheese (all types), cheese flavor, cream, curds, custard, ghee, hydrolysates (casein, milk protein, protein, whey, whey protein), ice cream, lactalbumin, lactalbumin phosphate, lactoglobulin, lactoferrin, lactulose, nou-

gat, pudding, rennet, rennet casein, Recaldent (used in teeth-whitening chewing gums), Simplesse, whey (in all forms), and yogurt. Milk can be found in margarines, breads, cookies, cakes, chewing gum, chocolates, caramels, cold cuts, crackers, cereals, nondairy products, processed and canned meats, and frozen and refrigerated soy products.

If a food is labeled "kosher pareve (or parve)," is it milk-free?

Just because a product is kosher, to be eaten as "nondairy" (pareve, or parve), does not mean it doesn't have some milk protein. In kosher labeling, a *D* on a product label next to the circled *K* or *U* indicates the presence of milk protein.

Does "nondairy" on a label mean the food is safe for people with a milk allergy?

No. There are products, such as nondairy creamers, that actually have milk ingredients. The label should include the term "milk," but seeing "nondairy" could be misleading. This is an example of why reading the entire ingredient label is necessary to avoid trouble.

What are some unexpected places where milk might be an ingredient or a contaminant?

Milk may be found in cosmetics, nutritional supplements, medicines, and pet foods. Deli meats could become contaminated with milk from cheeses cut on the same slicer. Sometimes fish or shellfish are "dunked" in milk or have milk protein added to reduce odors or change the consistency, so watch out for this practice and prefer fresh forms.

Do lactose-containing foods or medicines have milk protein in them?

Lactose is milk sugar and is not an allergen (not a protein). However, it is derived from milk. There are rare reports of lactose products triggering reactions in persons with milk allergy. In particular, residual milk protein in lactose used in some types of asthma inhalers triggered symptoms in exquisitely sensitive milk-allergic people.

If I have a milk allergy, can I use a medication in pill form that has lactose in it?
Pharmaceutical-grade lactose in oral medications has not triggered significant reports of reactions, possibly indicating a very low risk. It seems that lactose is usually free of milk proteins but may sometimes have a trace amount. If you wish to avoid the risk of trace contamination, formulations without lactose are usually possible to obtain. Often the liquid forms are lactose-free. You should investigate products individually and speak with your allergist about the risks.

Does cocoa butter or calcium lactate have milk?
You do not usually need to worry about cocoa butter, coconut milk, calcium lactate, oleoresin, or cream of tartar.

Is dark chocolate or cocoa safe for a person with a milk allergy?
Cocoa is a bean and a very uncommon allergen. Pure cocoa is safe for people with a milk allergy. Milk chocolate is clearly a problem for a person with a milk allergy, but many dark chocolates do not have milk ingredients and could be safe. However, studies have shown a very high rate of milk contamination in dark chocolate candy products, even some without advisory labeling ("may contain milk"). Therefore, I advise caution. Chocolates may be better purchased from specialty manufacturers that cater to people with food allergies (see the resources in chapter 11).

What formula can be given to a baby with milk allergy?
Over 90% of infants with milk allergy tolerate formulas approved as "hypoallergenic," specifically a type called an extensive casein hydrolysate. The formula is made of digested cow's milk protein. Most infants with cow's milk allergy will also tolerate soy, which has no relation to cow's milk but is in itself somewhat allergenic. A partially digested cow's milk–based formula, such as a partial whey hydrolysate, would not be a good choice because residual milk protein can trigger a reaction. If a hypoallergenic formula is not tolerated, a formula made from the building blocks of protein, amino acids, could be used. This type of formula, called an elemental formula, or amino acid–based formula, is expensive and poor tasting.

WHEAT AND OTHER GRAINS

Is wheat allergy the same as celiac disease?

Wheat allergy is different from celiac disease (also called sprue, or gluten-sensitive enteropathy). This is discussed more in chapter 5.

If I have a wheat allergy, what other grains can I eat?

Most people with a wheat allergy (about 80%) can tolerate other grains, such as barley and rye, although wheat contamination of other grains is sometimes a problem. Although you may need to check with your doctor before trying one, flour substitutes that are usually less allergenic include those made from amaranth, arrowroot, barley, buckwheat, corn, millet, oat, potato, rice, soybean, tapioca, and quinoa.

What terms on a label might indicate wheat, and what types of foods are often made of wheat?

Ingredients and foods of concern include bread crumbs, bulgur, cereal extract, couscous, durum (durum flour or wheat), emmer, einkorn, farina, flour (all-purpose, cake, enriched, graham, high gluten, high protein, pastry, wheat), Kamut (khorasan), semolina, spelt, sprouted wheat, triticale, vital gluten, wheat (bran, germ, gluten, malt, starch), and whole wheat berries. Expect to find wheat in ale, baking mixes, baked products, batter-fried foods, beer, breaded foods, breakfast cereals, candy, crackers, frankfurters and other processed meats, ice cream products, salad dressings, sauces, soups, soy sauce, and surimi.

What do I need to know about allergies to other grains?

Although it is possible to be allergic to any of the numerous grains and grain substitutes (amaranth, arrowroot, barley, buckwheat, corn, millet, oat, potato, rice, and quinoa), these are uncommon allergies. Those who are allergic to corn can usually have corn oil and corn syrup because they are not likely to have relevant amounts of protein.

Can a wheat-allergic person safely eat a communion wafer?

No. The wheat could trigger a reaction.

What communion wafer substitutes are available for a person with a wheat allergy?

For someone with a true wheat allergy, an entirely wheat-free substitute (such as a rice-based wafer) would be the safest option. There is a low gluten communion wafer, acceptable to the Vatican, for Catholics with celiac disease. The gluten content is 0.01%, which comes to 37 micrograms of gluten. The trace amount of wheat protein in the low gluten formulation carries a very small risk of inducing a reaction in a highly sensitive wheat-allergic person. Most people with a wheat allergy, however, would be able to tolerate this low amount, assuming the wheat content is accurate. A person could work with an allergist to determine through past reactions and possibly a medically supervised feeding whether the wafer would be safe. You should also check the full ingredients list for other allergens you are avoiding.

TREE NUTS

What foods are tree nuts?

The Food and Drug Administration (FDA) considers *a lot* of foods to be nuts. The main ones are almonds, macadamias, Brazil nuts, pecans, cashews, pine nuts (pignolia nuts), chestnuts, pistachios, filberts (hazelnuts), coconuts, and walnuts. Less common tree nuts that, according to U.S. law, must be disclosed in ingredients lists are beechnuts, butternuts, chinquapins, ginkgos, hickory nuts, lychee nuts, pili nuts, and shea nuts.

Are people with a tree nut allergy also allergic to peanuts?

People who are allergic to tree nuts are not necessarily allergic to peanuts (or vice versa), although there is increased risk because nuts are all more allergenic foods.

If you are allergic to one tree nut, are you allergic to all tree nuts?

People can be allergic to some tree nuts and not others, for example, allergic to walnuts but not cashews or almonds. However, some nuts have similar proteins—almonds and hazelnuts, pistachios and cashews, walnuts and pecans. Often a person has an allergy to both.

What is the relationship between cashews and mangoes?

Both are from the same food family (Anacardiaceae). The mango pit is allergenic, but not the pulp, which is the edible part. Therefore, having a cashew allergy does not mean there will be a problem eating mango pulp, although it is possible to be allergic to that part of the mango as well.

Is coconut a tree nut?

The FDA considers it a nut, but there is controversy. Most people see coconut as a fruit (a fibrous, one-seeded drupe).

If I have a tree nut allergy, can I eat coconut?

Coconut allergy is uncommon. Some coconut proteins are similar to those in walnuts, hazelnuts, lentils, and other foods, yet most people with allergies to these foods tolerate coconut. There are relatively few reports of coconut allergy in the literature, and a recent study of forty children with positive tests or known allergy to peanuts or tree nuts showed no increased risks for having positive tests or allergy to coconut. This is a situation where you should talk to your doctor unless you are already tolerating coconut. Coconut oil, probably containing little coconut protein to begin with, is low risk.

Is shea nut butter an allergen?

So far no allergic reactions to shea nut butter have been documented in the literature. In at least one study, no proteins could be detected in this derivative of shea nuts.

Is lychee (lichee) a nut?

The FDA includes lychee on its list of "nuts" requiring labeling disclosure, but it is actually a tropical and subtropical fruit. It is sometimes referred to as a "nut" when eaten in its dried form. Lychee is a rare allergen but, like most foods, has been reported to cause a severe allergic reaction in a few people. It has some allergenic relationships with pollens, latex, and sunflower seeds.

What foods might have nut ingredients?

Labeling laws require that a tree nut ingredient be named. Tree nut avoidance can be tricky because the nuts can be found in cereals, crackers, cookies, candy, chocolates, energy bars, flavored coffee, frozen desserts, marinades, barbeque sauces, some cold cuts (such as mortadella), gianduja (a creamy mixture of chocolate and chopped almonds and hazelnuts, although other nuts may be used), marzipan (almond paste), nougat, Nu-Nuts artificial nuts, Nutella, pesto, and nut meal. Some alcoholic beverages may contain nut flavorings. Natural extracts such as pure almond and wintergreen may have nut proteins (affecting the filbert / hazelnut allergy).

Which cuisines typically use tree nuts?

Tree nuts are common ingredients in foods from ethnic restaurants (such as Chinese, African, Indian, Thai, and Vietnamese), ice cream parlors, and bakeries.

What nonfood items could have tree nut ingredients?

Tree nut oils may be found in cosmetics, lotions and soaps, nutritional supplements, medications, and pet foods. Acorns are probably allergenic, but they are too sour for us to eat, so we will leave them for the squirrels.

Can I have artificial nut flavor if I am nut allergic?

Imitation and artificially flavored extracts are generally safe.

Is almond extract safe with an almond allergy?

Pure almond extract should be avoided because it likely has almond proteins. Peach or apricot pit extracts may also be used for making almond extract. Artificial and imitation almond extracts should be safe, although contacting the manufacturer is advisable. Alternatively, a different flavor, such as vanilla, could be substituted.

Can I have nut oils if I am allergic to tree nuts?

There can be a risk in eating these. Nut oils are not generally refined, so they do contain tree nut proteins.

Can I have nutmeg, water chestnuts, and butternut squash if I am nut allergic?
Although nutmeg, water chestnuts, and butternut squash have the word
"nut" in them, they are not peanuts or tree nuts. Nutmeg contains a chemical called myristicin, which in large amounts can induce dangerous toxic
effects and hallucinations. Although donuts also have the word "nut" in
them, you will need to consider the exact ingredients to know if they
really have any tree nuts in them!

If I am allergic to one nut, do I need to avoid all nuts?
A person may be allergic to one or two or many nuts. Avoiding all nuts
when there is an allergy to just one or two is a personal decision.

What are the risks of eating other nuts when there are allergies to some?
The risks include

- making a mistake in identification and eating the allergenic nuts
- getting exposed to the avoided nuts because of cross-contact with the
  nuts that are safe (if a walnut brownie also has cashews or pistachios,
  for example)
- becoming allergic to another kind of nut

How often do allergies develop to a nut that is already tolerated?
If a nut is already tolerated as a routine part of the diet, developing a new
allergy to it is uncommon.

*What considerations are important in deciding whether to eat some types of
nuts when there are allergies to other types?*
Some people decide to avoid all nuts to reduce their risk of accidentally
eating the ones they are avoiding. Others choose to eat the tolerated
nuts, being very careful about the foods they select. Because nuts are
often processed together, it is difficult to find ones that are not at risk for
cross-contact. Almonds are often selected as a tolerated nut to try because
they can be purchased in various forms without contamination by other
nuts. For example, specific brands of almond butter, almond milk, and
cereals are not processed with other nuts. The decision to eat some nuts

should be discussed with your doctor, for it involves considering risks (severity of allergy), dietary preferences, age, and other factors.

Can a person with a nut allergy eat hickory smoked foods?

Hickory smoking uses the wood from the hickory tree, not the nuts, and so there should be no risk.

SEEDS

What are examples of seeds?

There are many kinds of seeds, including sesame, sunflower, mustard, poppy, flax, pumpkin, and others.

If I am allergic to one seed, am I allergic to all seeds?

Allergy to one seed does not necessarily mean allergy to others.

Is it possible to tolerate eating a few seeds when eating more of that seed can trigger a reaction?

Yes. Since seeds are often used in small amounts in foods, people with seed allergies may have no problems because they never eat enough to cause symptoms. For example, sesame seeds on breads might be tolerated, but tahini, a paste that is primarily sesame protein, may trigger a reaction.

If I tolerate some sesame seeds on bread but react to larger amounts in tahini, do I need to avoid sesame on breads?

There are several issues to consider here. If a reaction to tahini was severe, you may be more motivated to completely avoid sesame in any form. If you routinely tolerate stray seeds, allowing them to remain in your diet may be less concerning. We do not know if eating a few seeds speeds, hinders, or has no effect on recovery from the allergy. A compromise may include not worrying about stray seeds but avoiding larger amounts. Clearly, decisions should be made in consultation with your allergist.

What seeds are most likely to cause allergy?

Sesame allergy is the most common seed allergy. Mustard and poppy seeds can also cause allergies, but these are comparatively uncommon.

If I have a sesame allergy, do I need to worry about allergies to other foods?

Sesame, like most foods, shares some proteins with other plants. For example, there is some relationship to peanuts, although most people with a peanut allergy tolerate sesame.

What products or ingredients may have sesame?

Sesame, and other seeds, is not currently included in U.S. labeling laws, although it is in many other countries. Food ingredients indicating sesame include sesame flour, sesame oil, sesame seeds, tahini (sesame paste), benne, and til or teel. Sesame is often in baked goods, bread crumbs, breads, rolls, bagels, crackers, breakfast cereals (such as granola, muesli, and Kashi brand cereals), dipping sauces and marinades, falafel, halvah, Japanese snack mix, protein and energy bars, sushi, tortilla chips, dips such as hummus and baba ghanoush, vegetarian "burgers," and herbal drinks, including Aqua Libra, a British herbal beverage.

Is sesame found in nonfood items?

Sesame may be found in, for example, cosmetics, nutritional supplements, medications, and pet foods. The scientific name for sesame, *Sesamum indicum*, might be on the label.

Is sesame oil safe for people with sesame allergies?

Sesame oil is usually not refined and therefore contains sesame proteins, so it is not safe.

SOY

If I have a soy allergy, can I eat peanuts and other beans?

Soy is a bean, yet most people with a peanut allergy are not allergic to soy.

People with a soy allergy may be able to eat peanuts, too, although the risk of being allergic to peanuts is increased if you are already allergic to soy.

What foods or terms on labels indicate soy?

Labeling laws require use of the term "soy" if it is an ingredient. Foods and words to look out for include edamame, miso, natto, shoyu sauce, soy (fiber, flour, grits, nuts, sprouts), soy substitutes (milk, yogurt, ice cream, cheese), soy protein (concentrate, hydrolyzed, isolate), soy sauce, tamari, tempeh, textured (or texturized) vegetable protein (TVP), and tofu (soybean curd). Soy is in many foods to add protein, such as baking mixes, breads, cookies, crackers, canned broth and soups, canned tuna and meat, breakfast cereals, high protein energy bars and snacks, low fat peanut butters, and processed meat, such as frankfurters. Asian restaurants are risky because soy is a frequent ingredient. Highly refined soy oil has no appreciable residual protein and is exempt from labeling, but it is often included on ingredient labels anyway.

Is soy found in nonfood items?

Soy may be found in cosmetics, nutritional supplements, medications, and pet foods.

I seem to tolerate soy but have reactions to soy protein isolate. Is that possible?

Yes. Soy protein isolate may have a concentrated amount of a particular protein from soy that is more allergenic for some people.

If I have reacted to soy protein isolate, do I need to avoid all soy?

The exact risks vary from person to person. Many people who react to soy protein isolate appear to tolerate other forms of soy, for example, soy flour in bread. It is often reasonable to continue eating the tolerated forms. However, your individual circumstances, particularly the severity of past reactions, should be discussed with an allergist. Soy protein isolate may be found in soy health food drinks, health bars, soups, hamburgers, and various other foods.

If I have a soy allergy, can I eat soy oil?
Yes. Soy oil is refined and is generally considered safe for people with soy allergy.

If I have a soy allergy, can I eat soy lecithin?
Most people with a soy allergy will tolerate foods that contain soy lecithin. This fatty derivative of soy has minimal protein and is used in low amounts in foods, often simply as a nonstick agent in baking.

Why do asthma medications that contain soy lecithin warn about soy and peanut allergies?
Although gradually leaving the market, some asthma inhalers have soy lecithin, a fatty derivative of soy with extremely low amounts of soy protein. Allergists often allow patients with a soy allergy to eat this derivative because it is rarely problematic. Therefore, despite the package warnings, the risk to soy-allergic people of an inhaled medication with soy lecithin is extremely low. The warning about a peanut allergy also seems overly cautious because not only is there almost no soy protein in soy lecithin to begin with, most people with a peanut allergy tolerate soy.

LEGUMES

What do I need to know about allergy to beans?
Among the numerous types of beans, peanuts and soybeans are the most common allergens. Allergies to chickpeas and lentils are described more often in Mediterranean countries.

If I am allergic to one bean, do I need to avoid all beans?
Usually not. It seems that among beans, peanuts and soy are the main culprits. There is a bean called lupine (lupin) that may be higher on the problem list than others, especially if someone already has a peanut allergy. Next in line are lentils, chickpeas, and green peas. Allergy to string beans, kidney, navy, lima, and others are far less common. A person with

an allergy to one bean can usually eat other beans, but a person who has had reactions to several beans might have trouble with most beans.

I tolerate canned beans but have reactions to raw ones. How is this possible?
Sometimes people are sensitive to pollen-related proteins in beans, which are destroyed by cooking or canning.

Are there hidden sources of legumes?
Legumes can be dried and used as a flour. Some pastas are fortified with beans such as chickpeas or lentils.

VEGETABLES AND STARCHES

What do I need to know about allergies to vegetables?
Countless vegetables have various botanical relationships to each other and to pollens. Many allergic reactions to vegetables are related to pollen allergies. People with allergies to pollen have mild allergic reactions to raw forms of a vegetable that has similar proteins to those in the pollen (see pollen-food allergy syndrome earlier in this chapter). Symptoms often vary depending on whether the food is cooked, which makes a reaction less likely to occur. Not all vegetable allergies can be tied to pollen allergies, however. People have also reported mild and, rarely, severe reactions to many vegetables without a clear connection to pollen allergies. Some of the more common culprits appear to be eggplants (actually a fruit), carrots, and celery.

Are some vegetables more allergenic than others?
It is very hard to find reports of allergies to broccoli, cauliflower, squash, cabbage, lettuce, mushrooms (fungus), sweet potatoes, olives, brussels sprouts, artichokes, or asparagus. Many other vegetables are more problematic than these, but reactions are still relatively uncommon. It is thought that some reactions, such as those to eggplant, may be caused by natural chemicals in the food that trigger allergy-like symptoms.

I can eat baked potatoes and French fries, but I sometimes get itchy from potato salad. Is that a sign of potato allergy?

Sometimes the potatoes used in potato salad are less cooked than other forms. Raw potatoes have residual proteins similar to those in birch pollens, whereas these proteins are destroyed when potatoes are cooked. In this case, the reaction may be to these proteins, assuming there is no allergy to other ingredients in the potato salad.

FRUITS

What fruits can cause allergic reactions?

There are countless fruits (berries, citrus, melons, pitted fruits, and so on) with many botanical relationships, and virtually all have caused a reaction in someone.

Are fruit allergies severe?

Most allergies to fruits are mild. Many reactions to fruits are related to a person having allergies to pollens and then experiencing mild allergic reactions, such as an itchy mouth, to raw forms of fruits with proteins related to the particular allergenic pollens (see pollen-food allergy syndrome discussed earlier in this chapter). Severe reactions to fruits are less common and are usually not related to pollen allergies.

Is it possible to be allergic to fruit seeds but not the fruit?

Yes, but this is rare. Reported reactions seem to be related to orange seeds in particular and may be more common in people with severe cashew or pistachio allergies.

MEATS

What meats cause allergies?
Allergies to any meats are overall uncommon but can occur with poultry meats (turkey, chicken, duck) and mammalian meats (beef, pork, lamb). Allergies to exotic meats (buffalo, horse, whale, kangaroo, and so on) are also possible.

If I am allergic to chicken, will I be allergic to eggs?
Having a chicken allergy does not usually mean you are at risk for an egg allergy.

If I am allergic to beef, will I be allergic to milk?
Cow's milk allergy is related to beef allergy, as described earlier in this chapter. However, it is possible to be allergic to beef without having a milk allergy.

Is it possible to be allergic to chicken and not turkey?
It is possible, but most people who are allergic to one type are reactive to both.

Does having a poultry allergy mean I'll have a mammalian meat allergy (or vice versa)?
No. Poultry allergies are different from mammalian meat allergies.

If I have an allergy to one type of mammalian meat, will I be allergic to others?
Having an allergy to beef likely means having an allergy to veal. Allergy to cow's meat may occur without allergy to other mammals, such as pork or lamb, but there is an increased risk. As in most foods, some proteins in meats are similar to ones in other substances (feather proteins, dog proteins, and so on), but this does not usually translate into problematic allergies.

I noticed allergic reactions many hours after eating mammalian meats. Is this possible?

There is an uncommon delayed reaction in some people, who develop typical allergic symptoms (hives, swelling, anaphylaxis) several hours after eating mammalian meats (pork, beef, lamb). People with this problem may also be at risk to react to certain cancer treatments that have a similar substance to meat. The reaction has been traced to complex sugars, rather than proteins, in the meats. People at risk appear to have been bitten by ticks, which somehow triggered the allergic response against the complex sugars in the muscle meats.

FISH

What are the different types of fish?

There are many types of fish, including anchovies, pike, bass, pollock, catfish, salmon, cod, scrod, flounder, swordfish, grouper, sole, haddock, snapper, hake, tilapia, herring, trout, mahi mahi, tuna, and perch. Fish is covered by U.S. labeling laws, which require that the type of fish be named.

If I am allergic to one type of fish, am I allergic to all types?

More than 50% of the time, an allergy to any type of finned fish means there is allergy to many types.

If I am allergic to one type of fish and perhaps not others, should I go ahead and eat the ones I can?

Since fish allergy can be severe, you have to be vigilant in avoiding triggers. You will need to take special care if you elect to eat some fish when others are a problem (because you may have a mix-up of fish or cross-contact during handling or cooking). This decision should be made in consultation with your allergist, discussing risks and preferences.

I can eat canned fish but not fresh fish. How is this possible?
Canned fish might be tolerated by a person who reacts to less heated forms because the canning process destroys some proteins.

Is it possible to be allergic to all seawater fish but not freshwater fish, or vice versa?
Fish allergy does not usually divide itself in that manner.

What is scombroid fish poisoning?
Spoiled dark-meat scombroid fish (marine fish such as mackerel, tuna, swordfish) can develop chemicals that are similar to histamine, the chemical released by immune cells during an allergic reaction. Eating the spoiled fish can result in symptoms that mimic an allergic reaction.

Is it possible to be allergic to some parts of a fish and not other parts?
Yes. Fish allergy can be very tricky. Allergies to some segments of fish and not others (for example, belly muscle versus side muscle) are not uncommon. For practical purposes, however, avoidance of the entire fish is typically advised.

Where might fish be found as a food or ingredient?
Fish can be an ingredient in unexpected places: Worcestershire sauce and Caesar salad and dressing usually contain fish (anchovies). Caponata, a Sicilian eggplant relish, may contain anchovies. Surimi, an artificial crabmeat (also known as "sea legs" or "sea sticks"), is made from fish. Fish proteins survive high heat, so if fish is made in a fryer, that fry oil can contaminate otherwise safe foods. Seafood restaurants are certainly high risk in general. Ethnic restaurants (such as Chinese, Indonesian, Thai, and Vietnamese) also use fish and fish ingredients in many dishes.

Is fish found in nonfood items?
Fish may be found in cosmetics, medicines, nutritional supplements (for example, omega-3 fatty acids), and pet foods.

If I have a fish allergy, can I use fish oil supplements?

Whether a worrisome amount of fish protein remains in omega-3 fatty acid supplements is unfortunately unclear (but the amount is probably exceedingly low). A discussion with your doctor about the risks is warranted, but alternatives (such as flax oil) are also available.

Can I eat carrageen if I have a fish allergy?

Carrageen is a marine algae, not a fish, and should be safe.

What is anisakis allergy and how is it related to fish?

Anisakis is a parasite (worm) that can inhabit fish such as herring, mackerel, and sardines and trigger an allergic reaction in someone who eats that fish, which would masquerade as an allergy to that fish. This problem is typically limited to countries where fish is eaten undercooked and never previously frozen.

Does having a fish allergy mean that I would be allergic to caviar?

No. However, some people are allergic to caviar.

Can I eat fish gelatin if I have a fish allergy?

No comprehensive studies have been done to determine whether relevant amounts of fish protein remain in fish-derived gelatin (kosher gelatin). If any proteins remain, the amounts are likely extremely low. Discuss with your allergist whether to avoid this gelatin.

SHELLFISH

What are the different types of shellfish?

Crustacean shellfish include lobster, shrimp, crab, prawns, crevettes, langoustine, crawfish, crayfish, and écrevisse. The non-crustacean types and other sea creatures include abalone, octopus, clam, scallop, cockle, snail (escargot), mussel, squid (calamari), and oyster.

If I am allergic to one type of shellfish, will I be allergic to all types?

Over 75% of people are allergic to all types of crustacean shellfish if they are allergic to any. The rate of allergy to non-crustacean shellfish and other sea creatures appears lower, but there is still a risk that would need to be addressed by your allergist. Non-crustacean shellfish are not included in U.S. allergen-labeling laws.

What foods or types of foods might have shellfish proteins?

Shellfish protein may be present in bouillabaisse, fish stock, surimi, and seafood flavoring (such as crab or clam extract). Fish and seafood restaurants are high risk, of course, even when nonshellfish menu items are ordered, because of cross-contact issues during processing and cooking.

Can I get radiocontrast dye if I have a shellfish allergy?

Yes. There is a myth that since there is iodide in radiocontrast dyes used for medical radiographic scans, like CAT scans, and iodide in shellfish, there is an allergic relationship. This myth stems in part from the misunderstanding that people develop food allergies to iodide, which isn't true. We eat iodide every day in salt. There are no shellfish proteins in radiocontrast dye. The most common reason people have allergic reactions to the dye is because the dye has a high salt concentration, which in some people triggers their allergy cells to release histamine. Although having a seafood allergy is not directly linked to radiocontrast dye allergy, it is true that people with allergies in general, including food allergies, may be at higher risk of also reacting to radiocontrast dye. Talk to your allergist. Usually a formulation with a lower concentration of salts is available, or those with a radiocontrast allergy can be premedicated to reduce risks.

Can I take glucosamine-chondroitin supplements if I have a shellfish allergy?

Glucosamine chondroitin is an over-the-counter dietary supplement that is derived from shrimp shell and shark cartilage. Presumably, the muscle proteins (which hold the allergens) would not contaminate the product, but this is currently uncertain. Talk to your doctor before trying these supplements.

Do people with shellfish allergy need to avoid chitosan and other chitin products?

Chitosan is derived from the chitin in the shells of shellfish. It is used in bandages, to help blood clot, in dietary supplements with various potential health claims, and in some industrial settings, such as for water filtration and pesticide use. One study evaluating ten people with shellfish allergy found no response to allergy skin testing with chitosan powder or bandages and no detectable shellfish proteins in the powder. Unfortunately, there is not much information on potential shellfish protein contamination of chitosan, but there is also no reported allergy despite widespread use. Thus, although some caution is warranted, the risk appears to be very low.

If I have a seafood allergy, can I take potassium iodide if there is a radiation emergency?

Yes. People might be given potassium iodide to protect their thyroid in the event of a nuclear emergency. Having a seafood allergy has nothing to do with an iodide allergy, so this treatment should be safe. Allergic reactions to iodide can occur, but these are not like anaphylaxis. Some people develop rashes from iodide-containing medical treatments (such as skin cleansers).

SPICES

What foods are spices?

Spices and other seasonings are derived from various plant materials, such as seeds, leaves, beans, fruit bodies, roots, or other plant parts. In general, spice allergies are uncommon, but when they occur, they are similar to those described for fruit, seed, and nut allergies, including the relationship to pollens. Among the spices, mustard is one of the more common allergens.

Is it possible to be allergic to multiple spices?
Yes. Some "spices" are actually combinations of more than one spice; for example, curry may have turmeric, cumin, pepper, and so forth.

How common are allergies to spices?
In general, they are uncommon, but they can be severe. When a person has an allergic reaction to a food and the triggering substance is unclear, I am always very interested in the exact ingredients, including spices.

Some spices make my nose run. Is that an allergy?
Some spices are spicy because they contain a chemical called capsaicin, which causes the "heat" in foods and may also trigger allergy-like symptoms, including redness and a runny nose. These are chemical and neurologic responses, not an allergic reaction.

ALCOHOLIC BEVERAGES

Is it possible to be allergic to or have allergic-like reactions to wine and spirits?
Yes, in several ways. Some people (particularly Asians) are unable to properly digest the alcohol. The by-products cause symptoms that can include skin redness, nausea, vomiting, sleepiness, and sometimes a wheeze. The same effect sometimes happens when alcohol and certain medications are being used at the same time. Some medications that affect how the body processes alcohol are the antibiotic metronidazole (Flagyl) and the antifungal medication griseofulvin (Fulvicin or Grifulvin). Drinking alcohol while using a skin cream called Elidel or Protopic causes a peculiar reaction in some people, who develop a redness where they applied the cream.

Sometimes wine has chemicals, like histamine, that may induce flushing and allergic symptoms. The sulfites in some wines, which are used as preservatives, cause symptoms in people who are sensitive to them, especially asthma symptoms. Some processing agents, such as egg used for clarification, might contribute allergens, but whether these are present in relevant amounts is unclear. Finally, wines and spirits can have allergens from the source ingredients (such as fruits, nuts, and grains).

What food proteins are in alcoholic beverages?

The relevance of residual food proteins in alcoholic beverages has not been extensively studied. As the beverage is made, some proteins may be altered in a way that reduces their allergenicity, but this possibility should not be relied on. Alcoholic beverages are derived from natural ingredients, so fruits, nuts, grains, spices, and other allergenic foods can be components of the beverage. Amaretto is derived from almonds, Frangelico from hazelnuts, and Irish cream from milk. Allergic reactions to beer are uncommon but appear to be related to residual grain proteins.

MISCELLANEOUS FOOD ALLERGENS AND COLORS, ADDITIVES, AND PRESERVATIVES

Babies are supposed to avoid honey. Is this a common allergen?

No. Although it is possible to be allergic to honey, the problem is rare. Babies are not supposed to ingest honey for a different reason. A bacteria in the honey could cause botulism, a type of neurologic problem, if ingested by children under a year of age.

Can people with insect sting allergies eat honey?

Yes.

What is a gelatin allergy?

Gelatin is derived from the skin and bone of beef, pork, or fish. It is an uncommon allergen. The way gelatin is processed may affect its potential to trigger a reaction in an allergic person. For example, gelatin in a soft, jiggly dessert may be less allergenic than gelatin in a chewy gummy candy. The ingredient is also used as a stabilizer in some vaccines, for example, the measles, mumps, and rubella (MMR) vaccine.

Can a person with a gelatin allergy eat beef or pork?

Usually. This is because the proteins causing the allergic reactions differ. However, people with delayed allergic reactions to beef or pork may be at slightly higher risk of gelatin allergy.

Can a person with an allergy to beef or pork gelatin eat fish gelatin?

Yes. There does not appear to be "cross-reactivity" between the mammalian-derived gelatin and the fish gelatin.

Can a person with a fish allergy eat fish gelatin?

This issue has not been adequately studied. It is not known if gelatin derived from fish (kosher gelatin) has trace residual fish proteins. The risk is likely low, but you should avoid it unless you consult with your allergist.

What unusual food or ingredients can a person be allergic to?

There are many! Almost anything eaten has caused an allergy in someone. Just a few examples. Caviar (fish egg) allergy can occur in people who tolerate fish. In China, allergies to bird's nest soup, made in part from saliva of a bird, have triggered reactions. Carmine is a food dye (red) that is derived from (get ready) the dried body of a beetle, and it has also triggered allergic reactions. Allergies to marijuana are also on record.

Do chemical additives and preservatives cause food allergies?

Yes, but much less often than ones derived from foods, and not in the same way, because the immune system does not respond to chemicals in the way it responds to proteins, which trigger typical allergies.

What natural, nonchemical food additives can cause allergic reactions?

Any additives that contain proteins can cause allergic reactions, although these allergies are rare. Examples include annatto, a yellow color derived from a seed, and saffron, from the dried parts of a flower, which is used for color and flavor. Other food additives that contain proteins are gelatin, gums from beans (such as tragacanth), and carmine dye (discussed above). Many foods also can be used to add color—beets, carrots, grape skins, paprika, turmeric, and so forth.

What is pectin?

Pectin is a gelling and thickening agent derived from fruits. Allergic reactions have been rarely described and seem to be a higher risk for persons with cashew or pistachio allergies (although most people with those nut allergies tolerate pectin).

What chemical food additives can cause adverse reactions?

Synthetic colors, preservatives, flavor enhancers, and curing agents are associated with some adverse reactions, but typically not allergic reactions.

What is tartrazine?

Tartrazine (yellow #5) is a synthetic color that has been investigated because of concerns that it may trigger hives, allergic reactions, and asthma.

Does tartrazine cause allergic reactions?

There are several reports of persons who developed nonallergic rashes from this colorant, such as occupational skin rashes. Despite many studies, a connection to asthma has not been proved and appears to be extremely rare, as are nasal reactions.

What are other examples of synthetic colors and are they related to allergy?

Many other synthetic colors (sunset yellow, erythrosine, ponceau 4R, carmoisine, quinoline yellow, patent blue, and others) have not been proved to cause allergic reactions. Some of these chemicals have been associated with illnesses on rare occasions (rashes, blood vessel disorders), but not typical allergic symptoms.

What is MSG?

MSG, or monosodium glutamate, is a flavor enhancer that occurs naturally in many foods and is used as an additive.

Does MSG cause allergic reactions?

The symptoms attributed to this additive, sometimes called the "Asian restaurant syndrome," include burning sensations, tingling, headaches, and drowsiness. Numerous well-designed studies have not been able to reproduce these symptoms routinely in persons believed to be affected. Very large doses, more than would be in typical meals, have reproduced some symptoms, but these are not thought to be allergic reactions.

What are parabens and benzoates?
Parabens and benzoates are preservatives that have been implicated in various allergic-type reactions, including anaphylaxis.

Do parabens and benzoates cause allergic reactions?
Studies suggest that these may rarely (in 2% to 3%) contribute to chronic hives. Benzoates have rarely been identified as a trigger of eczema. Anaphylaxis has been rarely reported.

Do BHA, BHT, nitrites, nitrates, sorbates, or aspartame cause allergic reactions?
There are several additives for which there appear to be a few documented cases of allergic-type reactions, but studies usually do not clearly implicate them. These additives include BHA and BHT (preservatives), nitrites and nitrates (curing agents), sorbates and sorbic acid (preservatives), and aspartame (sweetener). A few people have reportedly become sensitive to BHA through occupational exposure leading to skin rashes, with these rashes flaring when BHA was eaten. The take-home message is that allergic-type reactions to most additives are extremely rare and, if suspected, should be carefully evaluated further. Usually the suspicion will not be verified, thereby avoiding unnecessary restrictions.

What are sulfites?
Sulfites are added to foods as preservatives or anti-browning agents, or for a bleaching effect. Before 1986, sulfites were used more widely and in larger amounts, particularly on fresh foods such as lettuce.

What are symptoms of sulfite sensitivity?
Sulfites can induce asthma in sensitive persons. The asthma response is believed to be a chemical effect, not a typical allergic response. It seems that the more sulfite a food has, the more likely asthma could result from ingesting it.

What foods are high in sulfites?
Higher amounts of sulfites may be found in dried fruits, lemon juice, sauerkraut, wine vinegar, certain gravies, dried potatoes, and maraschino cherries, among other foods. Sulfites are declared on package labels.

Can sulfites cause nonasthmatic allergic reactions?
Despite a few reports of individuals who appear to have typical allergic reactions to sulfites (hives, anaphylaxis), well-designed studies usually do not confirm such reactions.

Are sulfites in medications a problem if I have sulfite sensitivity?
Sulfites are used to preserve some drugs and have been occasionally associated with triggering asthma. Epinephrine used to treat anaphylaxis has sulfites, but in low amounts that have never been reported to cause a problem (so epinephrine should never be withheld from a person sensitive to sulfites).

If I am sensitive to sulfites, can I use sulfa drugs?
Being sensitive to the preservative sulfite does not mean there is an allergy to medications that have sulfa.

WHEN TO SEEK HELP

See chapter 2 for more on this topic.

Why should I see a doctor for my or my child's food allergies?
It is essential to confirm a food allergy so that the correct foods are being avoided and a treatment plan is in place for any severe allergies.

When should I seek medical help for a suspicion of food allergy?
You should discuss your suspicions with your doctor as soon as possible.

Delving Deeper:
LATEX AND FOOD ALLERGIES

What does latex allergy have to do with food allergy?
Latex is derived from tree sap and therefore has natural proteins that are similar to some food proteins. However, because many foods have cross-reacting proteins, the relationships can be overwhelming to untangle and determine what foods might be allergenic to someone with latex allergy. Some latex-related troublemakers are bananas and kiwis. These two fruits have interrelationships with each other, pollens, and latex. Also related to latex allergy are chestnuts, avocados, mangoes, figs, peaches, tomatoes, potatoes, and bell peppers. These relationships are complex, and most people with an allergy to any one of these foods (or to latex) tolerate the others. If you do not already eat and tolerate the food related to your allergy, however, discuss with your doctor whether to avoid the food.

Also of Interest:
UNUSUAL FOOD REACTIONS

- Fixed rash from foods (the medical term is "fixed food eruption"). People with food allergy may develop a rash for several days in the same location each time they eat a particular food.

- Swelling from pressure on the skin associated with eating particular foods (the medical term is "food-related delayed-pressure urticaria and angioedema"). Delayed-pressure urticaria and angioedema is an illness where people develop swelling several hours after pressure is applied to the skin. In rare cases, this occurs only if the person ate a particular food.

- Body rashes from chemicals or metals in foods (the medical term is "systemic contact dermatitis"). Some people who develop itchy rashes when chemicals or metals are in direct contact with the skin may then develop widespread itchy rashes when they eat foods with the same substance (refer to the discussion of BHA reactions above). Nickel is a metal that can trigger skin sensitivity in some people. For example, they will gradually develop itchy rashes around nickel earrings or necklaces. The same individuals might react to nickel in the diet with itchy rashes in various places on the body. If you have this reaction, talk to your doctor about a nickel-free diet. It is not easy, and the effectiveness is somewhat controversial, but it involves letting tap water run before drinking to avoid leached metals; avoiding utensils with nickel in them and metal food containers and dispensers; and avoiding nickel-containing vitamins and medications as well as particular foods, including shellfish, all types of legumes, oatmeal, buckwheat, millet, lettuce, leavened breads, spinach, bran, cocoa, almonds, hazel, and licorice (this list is not comprehensive).

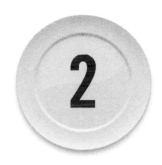

What Do I Need to Tell the Doctor to Help Get a
FOOD ALLERGY DIAGNOSIS?

This chapter answers questions about when and how to seek a food allergy diagnosis.

WHEN TO TALK TO YOUR DOCTOR

When should I suspect a food allergy?

If you or your child experience symptoms of allergy such as hives (like mosquito bites), rashes, swelling, itching, coughing, wheezing, or vomiting soon after eating a food, you should suspect a food allergy. There are also several chronic health problems that could be related to foods.

What chronic or persistent health problems are caused by food allergies?

Persistent skin rashes and chronic gut symptoms such as vomiting, pain, and diarrhea, perhaps with poor growth or weight loss, are sometimes associated with allergies to food.

When should I discuss my suspicion of food allergy with my doctor?

As soon as possible. You would not want to avoid a food that is not causing any problems, and you certainly would want to confirm any triggers so that you can remain healthy by avoiding them.

Why not self-diagnose a food allergy?
Usually when a person is suspicious of a food allergy, they are incorrect about the cause of their symptoms.

What type of doctor should I see if I suspect a food allergy?
You should start with your primary care doctor.

What does the internist, pediatrician, or family practice doctor do when evaluating a possible food allergy?
Your primary care doctor will need to consider if your symptoms are related to foods, to food allergy, or to another cause. This is important because many symptoms of food allergy can be explained by different allergies, by nonallergic responses to foods, or by a different illness altogether. Sometimes your primary care doctor will perform allergy testing and may refer you to an allergist for additional evaluation. Or, your doctor might run tests to determine common causes of your symptoms that are not related to having a food allergy.

Why see an allergist for food allergies?
An allergist, also called an allergist-immunologist, is a specialist who has received additional training in the diagnosis and management of food allergies and has access to additional tests to confirm or exclude an allergy.

HOW TO PREPARE FOR A DOCTOR VISIT

What should I do before seeing the doctor about a possible food allergy?
To help your doctor make a diagnosis, you should write down all details of the problems you have experienced. It is easy to get overwhelmed at a doctor's visit, and having things written down can be helpful. Record the symptoms, how long you have had them, their timing in relation to any foods, and the details about your diet that may inform your doctor of possible triggers. Prepare a diet record (see below). Also, bring in ingredient labels of foods that you suspect to be a problem and perhaps some that you routinely tolerate.

Your doctor may have a medical questionnaire for you to complete as well.

It is also helpful to prepare a list of questions you have about possible food allergies, but you will likely have many of those questions answered by this book!

What key questions should I ask my doctor?

Aside from determining if you have a food allergy, be prepared to ask these important questions. Is this severe? What foods do I need to avoid? How do I avoid these foods? Do I need emergency medications? How do I use those medications? Should I see an allergy specialist? What follow-up is needed?

What is a diet record?

A diet record shows what you are eating, when, and any symptoms. You can record this on lined paper. Write down all the ingredients of foods and beverages, what you were doing at the time you experienced symptoms (exercise, resting, etc.), and any medications you were taking. If the symptoms are repetitive or chronic, it is helpful to include meals that you seem to tolerate. You may wish to record several days of typical meals and symptoms.

Why should I keep a diet record?

If it is not clear what triggered your symptoms, you and your doctor can review the relationship to specific meals. The allergenic food will usually trigger symptoms each time it is eaten, so the diet record may help to narrow the possibilities. Make sure all the ingredients are listed, especially for meals that triggered symptoms.

Are there ways to narrow down which foods might be causing symptoms?

Remember that foods eaten often without symptoms are not as likely to be triggers as the accidental inclusion of a known allergen (a nut, for example, when you already know you have tree nut allergies) or a new allergy to an ingredient that you do not commonly ingest (for example, some spice that you do not eat often).

Are there circumstances around the time of a meal that could cause me to have a reaction to a food I usually tolerate?

Absolutely. If you have a reaction that seems to be to a food you usually tolerate, you should think about different variables. Did you eat more of something than usual? Were you taking any medications, including over-the-counter ones? Did you exercise after the meal? Did you have alcohol with the meal? Were you ill, with fever? Were you menstruating? These additional circumstances sometimes enhance the response to a potential food allergen.

What is the value of bringing ingredient labels?

Sometimes a minor or hidden ingredient is the cause of a reaction. Having the ingredient label on hand may help to identify an otherwise unsuspected trigger.

How do I obtain ingredient information from manufacturers?

Most ingredients will be listed on a label. However, sometimes vague terms are used to hide proprietary ingredients. For example, terms such as "spices" or "flavors" may be used. You can contact a manufacturer to try to get those "secrets," but it may be difficult. You may wish to see what your doctor thinks about the possibility of a hidden ingredient being the trigger, then work together to obtain more information from the manufacturer if needed.

How do I obtain ingredient information from a restaurant?

Discuss the ingredients in a nonaccusatory manner. Explain that you are concerned about a food allergy and want to consider any possible ingredients. If you have a known allergy and have a reaction at a restaurant, inform the restaurant promptly and discuss the preparation to determine whether the reaction could have been to accidental inclusion of your known trigger(s) or to another ingredient that may be a new problem.

Would I need to be off any medications prior to the office visit?

For your first visit with your primary care doctor, you do not likely need to avoid any medications. An allergist may request that you avoid antihistamines and some other medications that may block results to allergy skin testing. Asthma medications and most other medications can be continued.

Should I bring suspect foods with me to the doctor visit?
Especially if you are seeing an allergist, you may want to bring any unusual ingredients that were in the meal that triggered a reaction or that you suspect may be an allergen. The allergist may use that food to perform a skin test.

If I had a reaction to a packaged food or restaurant meal, should I bring that to the visit?
If it is not clear what triggered the reaction, it may be helpful to bring the actual foods, along with any ingredient lists or labels. Wrap the foods and label them "DO NOT EAT," then freeze them until the allergy visit.

Should I bring medications with me to the visit?
You should always bring all your medications to the visit. This allows your doctor to accurately review them and provides an opportunity to review your technique of use, for example, for nasal sprays and asthma inhalers.

What medical records should I bring to a visit to discuss possible food allergies?
When you are seeing a new doctor, you should bring relevant records from any previous doctor visits. An allergist is often interested in any prior allergy tests that were performed.

What will the doctor do during the visit to evaluate for food allergy?
The doctor should take a careful medical history, perform a physical examination, and consider any testing, if needed.

What is the doctor looking for in the medical history?
The medical history is crucial for the physician to consider if food allergy is the correct diagnosis or to determine an alternative one. The doctor will consider whether the symptoms are typical of allergy, are related to

specific foods, or have alternative explanations. All these clues are in the discussion you have with the doctor and any records you may have.

What is the doctor looking for during the physical examination?
Sometimes there are rashes or other physical evidence of allergy or of illnesses that may provide an alternative explanation for the symptoms.

What tests might the doctor perform?
A primary care doctor may perform a blood test. An allergist may perform blood tests as well as allergy skin tests and other tests. These and others are explained in detail in chapter 3.

FINDING THE RIGHT DOCTOR AND OTHER HEALTH PROFESSIONALS

How do I find a doctor who cares for people with food allergy?
A board-certified allergist-immunologist is specifically trained to diagnose and treat food allergies. You may discuss a referral with your primary care doctor. You can also search for doctors near you by zip code on www .aaaai.org, the website for the American Academy of Allergy, Asthma, and Immunology, or on www.acaai.org, the website for the American College of Allergy, Asthma, and Immunology.

What qualifications should I look for in an allergist to treat my food allergies?
As you would want from any doctor, the allergist should be compassionate, ready to listen carefully to your concerns, and willing to explain diagnosis and treatment to your satisfaction. Friends or relatives may have advice on a good doctor. I recommend seeing an allergist who is board-certified by the American Board of Allergy and Immunology (or a similar certifying board outside the United States).

What is a board-certified allergist-immunologist?
This certification is given to a physician who was initially trained and

certified to be a pediatrician, internist, or both, and has completed an additional two to three years of training in a fellowship learning the care of allergic disorders, including asthma, hay fever, anaphylaxis, food allergy, insect sting allergy, and immune system problems. Certification requires passing a final test, and maintaining the certification requires ongoing educational activities and periodic retesting.

How do I determine if my allergist is board-certified?
You can check on the website of the American Board of Allergy and Immunology at www.abai.org.

What other health professionals care for food allergy?
A gastroenterologist may be helpful in the care of chronic gut symptoms related to food allergies. A registered dietitian may be helpful in treatment.

Why would I see a dietitian?
When foods are removed from the diet due to allergies, there could be nutritional deficits. A registered dietitian can evaluate the diet to ensure that proper substitutes or supplements are providing appropriate nutrition. The dietitian can also provide advice regarding food allergen avoidance.

What is the difference between a dietitian, a nutritionist, and a dietetic technician?
They have different training and expertise. Whatever specialist you choose, it can be helpful to discuss their experience with food allergies. If your child is the patient, confirm the practitioner's experience with pediatric concerns.

What is a registered dietitian?
A registered dietitian (R.D.) has earned a bachelor's degree, completed an accredited practice program, passed a qualifying examination, and is required to continue educational activities to maintain certification. The degree indicates expertise in food and nutrition. Some registered dietitians may also refer to themselves as nutritionists.

What is a nutritionist?

A person taking the title of nutritionist may have forms of training that differ from those of a registered dietitian, with varying types of certification based on the state.

What is a registered dietetic technician?

A registered dietetic technician has earned a two-year associate's degree and completed 450 hours of supervised practice (about half the hours of an R.D.).

What about seeing a naturalist, alternative medicine practitioner, or acupuncturist?

Several nontraditional practitioners address food allergies. Many people pursue such evaluation and treatment, but the methods employed are often unproved or even disproved. Remember, if a treatment were valid and proved, it would be widely used. Exploring these alternatives is a buyer-beware situation, and it is advisable to pursue traditional medical evaluations and treatments as well. Unproven and disproven methods are reviewed in chapter 3.

Delving Deeper:
ALTERNATIVE THERAPIES

How often do people seek alternative therapies for food allergies?

In a survey study that my group performed among 380 families attending conferences about food allergies, 22% had tried alternative forms of diagnostic testing (which are considered unproved) such as serum IgG4, electrodermal skin testing, and muscle strength testing. Alternative therapies had been tried by 18%.

What alternative medicine practitioners treat food allergy?

Participants in my study used several types of complementary and alternative medicine practitioners, the most common being chiropractors, homeopaths, and acupuncturists. Only 49% of patients using these practitioners and therapies disclosed this to their physicians.

Among the people in your study who had tried alternative therapies, what was the overall opinion of these treatments?

Efficacy ratings for the treatments were poor, but the study participants overall expressed a preference for herbal therapy. When asked what they would choose if they could get an herbal treatment of equal efficacy, safety, and cost to a pharmaceutical drug, three times as many people with a preference preferred an herbal treatment. This tells me that people believe that natural or herbal treatments are, for some reason, better. My concern is that the safety of existing herbal treatments has often not been investigated. Being "natural" does not make a treatment safe.

Are there any dangers to alternative therapies for food allergy?

I do not have a strong feeling against people trying alternative means. I also understand people wanting to investigate treatment options, but I do worry about problems that could arise. For example, abandoning routine treatment could lead to a bad outcome while emphasis is directed to another therapy that is unproved. Practitioners of many alternative therapies are not monitored. Unproven treatments, even when they are "natural," could have side effects. In fact, there is an apparent misconception that alternative therapies are automatically safer than standard Western pharmaceutical approaches. It should be appreciated that many medications we routinely use today were initially derived from plants. They differ from alternative remedies primarily in that standard medications are typically well studied, side effects are known, and manufacturing is standardized. Herbal products in the United States are not regulated, ingredients can vary, and the products can remain on shelves as long as they are not proved unsafe. Nonetheless, it is possible to have side effects from herbal treatments, including allergic reactions. Overall, natural remedies are a constant buyer-beware situation.

Also of Interest:
TESTS TO AVOID

What food allergy tests should I avoid?

Many tests that are purported to be useful to diagnose food or other allergies are unproved. The rationale behind some of these tests can be quite convincing to people without a medical background. For example, cytotoxic testing, which is a blood test performed by mixing the food with blood cells and monitoring the cells, seems plausible. Other tests seem clearly implausible, such as analyzing hair (which is dead) or checking a pulse. The various unproven and disproven tests are discussed in chapter 3. When you are initially being evaluated for food allergy, I suggest seeing a board-certified allergist who performs traditional tests rather than taking a chance on the unproven ones. It is also helpful to look up specific tests and treatments on the website maintained by Dr. Stephen Barrett, appropriately titled Quackwatch (www.quackwatch.com).

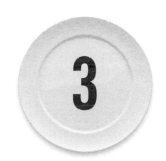

These Food
ALLERGY TESTS
Are Confusing!
What Do They Mean?

This chapter answers questions about allergy tests, explaining how they are selected and interpreted.

GENERAL QUESTIONS ABOUT TESTING

What is the most important test to diagnose a food allergy?

The medical history. Although not often thought of as a "test," this is much more important than any blood or skin tests for allergy.

Why is the medical history so important for diagnosing a food allergy?

As described in chapter 2, your doctor needs to know details about symptoms and diet to determine if food allergy is a possibility as well as to decide if additional tests are needed and which tests to perform. The tests are only helpful when they are interpreted in the context of the medical history.

Can a food allergy be diagnosed by medical history alone?

Sometimes the medical history makes a diagnosis obvious. For example, if a person repeatedly develops severe allergy symptoms minutes after eating a particular food, a diagnosis of allergy to that food is evident. Nonetheless, experts recommend a confirmatory test.

What tests are used to diagnose a food allergy?
Allergy skin tests and blood tests are most often used. These tests detect IgE antibodies, the immune system protein that causes many types of allergic reactions to foods, as described in chapter 1. Additional tests are elimination diets and feeding tests.

How are allergy tests used to diagnose a food allergy?
Skin and blood tests are selected and interpreted in the context of the medical history to provide additional evidence for or against an allergy to a specific food. Feeding tests give the most definitive evidence about a food allergy.

What foods can be tested?
Essentially any foods can be tested. Companies make extracts for skin testing and blood tests for many foods. Not all foods have commercial tests, however. As described below, an allergist may be able to create a test using the food itself.

Are there tests for dyes, preservatives, and food colors?
Although tests can be made for these substances, reactions to them, as described in chapter 2, are generally not caused by IgE unless the trigger has proteins (that is, an additive derived from a natural substance, like a seed).

SKIN TESTS

What are allergy skin tests?
An allergy skin test is a quick and simple way to determine if the body has made IgE antibodies to the food being tested.

How are allergy skin tests performed?

A small amount of liquid extract of the food being tested is introduced into the top layer of skin using a metal or plastic probe to scratch the skin surface. Because the skin is scratched, or "pricked," these tests are often called scratch tests or prick skin tests. In addition to the foods being tested, salt water and histamine tests are placed.

Where are the skin tests placed?

The tests are placed on a rash-free area of the less hairy part of the forearm or back.

What foods can be tested by skin tests?

Commercial extracts of over a hundred foods are approved for testing. An allergist can also make tests from whole fresh foods.

Why are fresh raw or whole foods sometimes used for allergy skin tests?

Commercially prepared extracts are most often used to test for food allergies. Sometimes an unusual food without a commercial extract must be tested, so allergists make their own extracts. Sometimes the commercial extract is missing some proteins that were lost in processing or storage, and the doctor may elect to use a fresh extract to avoid missing a diagnosis if the medical history indicates a possible allergy.

What does a positive test look like?

Like a mosquito bite. There is a raised center and surrounding redness. When positive, the raised center is usually between the width of a pea and a nickel.

Why is a histamine skin test performed while doing food skin tests?

Histamine is a chemical released from allergy cells that causes symptoms such as itching, swelling, and redness. The histamine skin test result should be positive, showing that the tests were reliable and not suppressed by any medications. The test represents an average positive for comparison. The histamine in the test is manufactured; it is not from people.

Why is a salt water skin test performed while doing food skin tests?

Salt water produces a negative result for comparison. No one is allergic to salt water (saline), but some people develop swelling just from the skin irritation of being scratched. This test allows the doctor to take this non-specific irritation response into account when evaluating the food tests.

What are the food allergy skin tests measuring?

IgE antibodies to the food that was tested. A positive test occurs when a person's immune system has made IgE antibodies that recognize the proteins in the test. If this is the case, doctors say that the person is "sensitized" to the tested food.

At what age can skin tests be performed?

Any age. Even infants can be tested.

Are the food allergy skin tests accurate in infants and young children?

They are helpful at any age; however, infants are slightly more likely to register a negative test despite having an allergy.

Do the skin tests hurt?

No. Most people feel a slight discomfort during the scratch, similar to a fingernail scratching the skin. There is no bleeding. The positive tests become itchy, but this is usually mild and goes away quickly.

Is there anything I can do to make the tests less uncomfortable?

Most infants do not cry because the discomfort is minimal. Children may be more likely to cry because of fear, so addressing this is helpful. Distracting a child with a song, video, story, or other means may lessen the anxiety. After the doctor reads the results, a cool compress may be soothing, but this is often not necessary. If there is significant itching, an antihistamine can be taken or a cream applied.

How long until a result is obtained from the skin test?

Positive tests may begin to show in minutes. They are read by the doctor at 10 to 20 minutes.

What should I do while the tests are developing?

Don't scratch! Rubbing the test could affect the results. Children may be kept busy with a game or other distraction. It is okay to roll down sleeves or put a shirt back on to cover the tests as they are developing.

How does the doctor record the skin test result?

The size of the bump in the middle of the response is measured. Doctors may record the size in various ways and may also measure the redness surrounding the bump. The bump is called a wheal, and the redness is called the flare.

How long before the skin test bumps go away?

The itching usually subsides in about 10 to 20 minutes, and the bumps generally fade within an hour, although sometimes they last much longer, depending on their size.

Can the skin test bumps come back?

Rarely, a bump reappears a few hours later only to fade again.

Can skin tests cause allergic reactions?

When positive, the test is causing a small, local allergic reaction on the skin surface just where the scratch was made. Since allergens are being scratched into the skin, there is a very small risk of an allergic reaction beyond the spot that was pricked.

What type of allergic reaction might occur from the skin tests?

If there is any allergic reaction beyond the expected bump, it is usually just a hive or two near the one caused by the test. It is very unusual to have more of a reaction than that.

What is the risk of a severe reaction from skin testing?

Allergic reactions such as nasal symptoms or spreading hives or a more severe reaction happen in fewer than one in a thousand people being tested and are usually associated with having large numbers of tests at once with many of them registering positive.

Are there situations when skin tests cannot be done?
Sometimes with extensive rashes, there is nowhere to put the test.

Are there situations when skin tests should not be done?
If antihistamines have been used recently, the tests can be blocked, and testing should be postponed.

Is it okay to do a skin test to a food that caused severe anaphylaxis?
If there is a recent history of severe anaphylaxis and one specific food was clearly the cause, many allergists will opt to use a blood test rather than a skin test for confirmation because the skin test will likely be positive and the reaction may be larger and more uncomfortable. However, it would not be wrong to go forward with a skin test to obtain quick confirmation of the allergy.

Can skin tests cause a food allergy?
Experts do not think so. No comprehensive studies confirm this conclusion, but many factors suggest this is not a concern. Individuals test negative in multiple years, those with positive tests often tolerate the foods, tests become negative over years of repeated testing, the food is introduced only to the top layer of the skin in small amounts, and emerging studies are suggesting that the skin may be a route to consider for treatment of food allergy.

Do I need to stop taking any medications to prepare for having skin tests?
Yes, you need to stop taking antihistamines for a period before the tests. The newer nose sprays with antihistamines may also need to be stopped. You can continue most other medications, including those for asthma, hay fever, and eczema. However, some medications that are not antihistamines may affect the tests, such as some antidepressants, so talk to your doctor.

How long do I need to avoid antihistamines or other medications for skin testing?
Different types of antihistamines last longer than others in the body, and

there is also variability from person to person. Check with your allergist. In general, four days off is adequate for Benadryl, diphenhydramine, chlorpheniramine, and brompheniramine; one week for Atarax, Zyrtec, Clarinex, hydroxyzine, Allegra, Rynatan, and Vistaril; and 10 days for doxepin and Periactin. Sometimes you can switch from a longer-acting antihistamine to a shorter-acting one, so medications can be used closer to the visit date. For example, switching from Allegra to Benadryl a week before and then stopping the Benadryl four days before would be an option, but be careful about the sedating effects of shorter-acting antihistamines, for example if driving.

Is there a way for the allergist to check if I have been off antihistamines long enough to be tested?

Yes. If you are not sure, the allergist can begin by placing just a histamine test. If this test causes a sufficiently large response, the remainder of the planned tests can be placed. Otherwise, testing would be postponed.

What do I do if I need an avoided medication before an appointment for skin testing?

Take it. Your allergist may be able to perform blood tests instead because these are not affected by the antihistamines, or you can reschedule the skin tests. A single dose may not interrupt the tests, so call ahead and explain what you took and when.

How many skin tests should be done?

There is no exact answer to this question because tests should be selected based on suspicions about which foods might be causing symptoms. Usually only a few foods are being considered as potential triggers at any one time, so selection of relevant foods is unlikely to require more than 10 to 15 tests.

Should I be tested to every food to see what I might be allergic to?

There is certainly no reason to test any foods already in the diet that are not causing any symptoms. Also, the tests have limited accuracy, so they do not give definitive "yes or no" results. For these and other reasons, your doctor should select foods that make sense as potential allergens warranting a test.

What does a positive or negative skin test mean?
A positive test means that the body has made IgE antibodies that recognize the protein in the test. This is called being sensitized. A negative test means that no such IgE has been detected.

Is a person ever able to eat the food anyway after a positive skin test?
Yes, yes, and YES!

Why can some people eat the food anyway despite a positive skin test?
The skin test detects that the immune system has made IgE antibodies to a food, but having IgE antibodies to a food often happens in people who are nonetheless able to eat the food. This is why the medical history is so crucial for proper test selection and interpretation.

Can a skin test be negative and a person still be allergic?
Yes, but not often.

Why would a skin test be negative in a person who is actually allergic?
Four reasons. First, although uncommon, the extract may be missing a relevant protein for the individual. Foods are made of many different proteins, and some of them may be under-represented in a test. In this case, if suspicion is high, another test could be performed, such as a skin test with fresh, raw food or a blood test. Second, the person may have a type of allergy that is not caused by IgE antibodies, so the test result is not relevant. Third, the use of antihistamines may have blocked the result, although this would likely have also blocked the histamine comparison test. And fourth, there could have been human error, in which case the test can be repeated.

Are the skin tests accurate?
Yes. They are excellent for detecting IgE antibodies to the protein being tested. But they must be interpreted in the context of the medical history, because a positive test alone does not prove a true allergy.

What would be an example of using a test result and a history together to diagnose a food allergy?

Let's suppose you had an itchy mouth during a meal in which sesame and mustard were the only foods you did not routinely eat. If the sesame test was positive and the mustard test was negative, then the evidence is strongest that the sesame was the culprit. But if you were tested to wheat, which was also in the meal, and it was positive, that would not diagnose a wheat allergy because you eat wheat all the time without a problem—that wheat test should not even have been performed.

Why are the skin test bumps measured or "graded" in size?

The larger the bump, or wheal, the more likely the food tested is truly a problem.

Do skin tests predict the severity of an allergy?

No.

Why would skin wheal size not reflect the severity of an allergy?

The larger the wheal, the more likely the food tested is actually a problem. However, multiple factors influence severity. The allergy test does not know if you have asthma (associated with more severe reactions), how much of the food you might have eaten (the more eaten, the worse a reaction might be), or your state of health at the time of an allergic reaction. This is why the wheal size is not a good predictor of an allergy's severity.

BLOOD TESTS (AND HOW THEY COMPARE WITH SKIN TESTS)

What blood tests are available for food allergy testing?

There are commercial blood tests for allergy to well over a hundred different foods.

What are the food allergy blood tests measuring?

IgE antibodies that the immune system has made against the proteins of foods in the test.

Why does a doctor perform a blood test for food allergy?
To determine whether, and how much, food-specific IgE antibodies are in the bloodstream.

What does a positive or negative blood test mean?
A positive test indicates the presence of IgE antibodies to the tested food, and a negative test indicates that the test did not detect these antibodies.

How are blood test results reported?
The test might be reported as classes, counts, or units.

Why do blood test results get reported in different ways?
The different methods of reporting have to do with tradition and technical aspects of the test. Nowadays an increasing number of laboratories are reporting the results in units called kIU/L or kUa/L.

What does kU/L or kUa/L mean?
It stands for a measure of units per liter. This is similar to a concentration, such as how much of something is in a specified space. In this case it is the amount of IgE that is specific to the food allergen. In this format, the test runs from "undetectable," usually signified by <0.35 or sometimes <0.10, to a high of >100. The < symbol means "less than," and the > symbol means "greater than."

Can blood test results from different laboratories be compared to each other?
It depends. If laboratories are using the same approved, automated test system for all your tests, the results can be compared. However, there are three test systems in use. Each of the three manufacturers creates its food test in a slightly different way, so results from one system's manufacturer may not be exactly the same as those from another. Your doctor should know which test system the laboratories are using.

Can a blood test be positive and not indicate a food allergy?
Yes. The test accurately measures IgE antibodies to the food, but a person can have IgE antibodies to a food and tolerate eating the food anyway.

If a blood test is negative, can there still be a food allergy?

Yes. This can occur because either the type of allergy being evaluated does not depend on IgE antibodies, or the proteins from the food in the test did not include ones that are relevant to the particular individual. Rarely, there can be a laboratory error as well. When results do not make sense, the test might be repeated, or another test, such as the skin test, might be performed.

What is an example of when a blood test was negative but there was an allergy anyway?

A patient who had a severe reaction to bananas had negative skin and blood tests to bananas. However, she clearly had symptoms that were severe when she was eating a banana, and no other foods or explanations made sense. When she was skin tested using a bit of raw banana, the test was positive. This confirmed her allergy and suggested that the previous tests had been negative because she was sensitive to a protein primarily present in the raw preparation. The extracts and blood test missed that protein for this patient.

What does a higher blood test result mean?

The higher the result, the stronger the positive test and the more likely a true food allergy is present.

Can a blood test for allergy be so strongly positive that it confirms a definite allergy?

In some circumstances, yes. Studies in children, using the Phadia Immu-noCAP brand test (now called the Thermo Fisher ImmunoCAP), have showed that almost all children with particularly high test results had true allergies. The general conclusion was that most of the young children who tested over 6 kIU/L for egg or 15 kIU/L for milk or peanut had a reaction. However, this minimum value of kIU/L where a child reacts varies by the child's age and allergic illness, the type of food, and other factors. There are only a few studies relating allergy outcomes to the test results, and the results differ, so the numbers quoted above may not always apply. Most foods have not been adequately studied, nor have the various manufacturers' tests. Therefore, it is important for allergists to interpret each test in light of individual circumstances.

How does the relationship between a test result and a food vary by age?

Based on limited studies, specific values seem related to higher risk for younger children. For example, a test result of 2 kIU/L for a 1-year-old may be high and associated with a strong risk of allergy while the same result may be unlikely to indicate an allergy in a 10-year-old. The relationship has not been studied into adulthood.

Is there a low positive blood test result that guarantees there is no allergy to the food?

Although lower test results are more favorable indicators that a food will be tolerated, no results by themselves are definitive to exclude an allergy. However, if the medical history is not compelling and the test is negative, this usually excludes the food as a trigger.

How are the blood tests different from the skin tests?

The tests are more similar than different. They both measure IgE antibodies to the food being tested.

Which is more accurate, skin or blood tests?

Both tests are excellent at detecting even small amounts of food-specific IgE antibodies. Sometimes one test will be positive while the other is negative.

Why does the accuracy differ among tests?

The tests are made by extracting proteins from the foods. Each food is a collection of many different proteins, and an individual with an allergy may be reacting to any of them. Different manufacturers of skin test extracts and of the blood tests use different techniques to extract the proteins. There may be subtle differences in the amount and types of proteins from one particular food that each test can measure. Therefore, sometimes the test results differ, favoring either a skin or a blood test.

How does a doctor decide whether to do the skin test, the blood test, or both?
Both tests give similar information, but a doctor selects one, the other, or
both based on medical circumstances. Often, the skin test is performed
when an immediate result is desired or an unexpected result occurred
from a blood test. The blood test is often used to monitor an allergy over
time because it is easier to compare results from one year to the next with
a blood test than it is with a skin test.

What is an example of why you might pick one test in particular?
Let's consider a child who, according to her mother, had a rash flare twice
when eating eggs. I assume that the child does have an egg allergy because
the story is consistent, and I am interested in monitoring the allergy over
time. I send a blood test to the lab, and it comes back showing undetectable, <0.35 kIU/L. This is a surprise, so I have the family return. The
mother now wonders if maybe something else was in the food, for example, cinnamon. I skin test to egg and to cinnamon, and only the egg test
is positive. This is an example where the skin test was a bit more sensitive
than the blood test, and indeed it was an egg allergy all along.

Do I need to avoid any medications before having the blood tests?
No.

How many foods can be tested in the blood test?
It is conceivable to order many dozens of tests, but this is usually not necessary. Tests should be selected based on the medical history, and usually
this means testing fewer than a dozen foods. The number of foods that
could be tested are limited only by the amount of blood taken.

What are food allergy "panel" tests?
To make testing convenient, manufacturers create panels of tests, so a
doctor can check a box and obtain groups of tests, rather than indicating
each food separately. These panels might be for common food allergens,
such as eggs, milk, peanuts, wheat, and soy. Or they might represent
groups of foods, such as tree nuts.

Should I be tested to a panel of "everything"?

No. Because tests are not able to diagnose an allergy by themselves, it is not a good idea to indiscriminately have dozens or even hundreds of tests performed. Many tests will be positive for foods that are actually completely innocent and tolerated components in the diet, and these positives can be misleading.

Should I be tested to a panel of foods that are related to one that caused an allergy?

It depends. Considering your medical history and understanding the relationships of foods is the first step. For a person allergic to peanuts, a bean, positive test results for other beans, such as soy, pea, and string bean, is common (over 50%), but true allergy to the other beans occurs in only about 5% of people with peanut allergies. In this situation, testing to a panel of beans could give misleading positive results. Test selection must be based in part on what the person is already eating and tolerating and what the person may not have eaten and may be at risk for, among other factors.

Why would a doctor decide to test me to a panel of foods?

Unfortunately, sometimes doctors inappropriately use test panels for convenience. Rather than picking the needed tests individually, they might just send a preselected "panel" to save time. Although this approach is not unreasonable, it can create confusion and anxiety when results are positive to foods that are otherwise of no concern. In some cases, however, panels of tests are appropriate to screen for possible allergy. An example would be a young child who reacted to a single tree nut but has not tried to ingest any other tree nuts. In this case, an allergist might order a panel of tests to tree nuts to determine which among the group could pose a risk.

Why would a doctor decide not to test me to a panel of foods?

There is really no reason to test for a food that is already tolerated in the diet and for which there is no concern of allergy. For example, testing a panel that includes milk, egg, soy, and wheat is not necessary for a person already eating those foods without any symptoms or chronic illnesses raising suspicions of allergy to those foods.

Does the blood test predict the severity of an allergy?
No. At least not very well. A few studies suggest that people with a higher test result might be more prone to severe reactions, but other studies do not show this pattern.

Why wouldn't a blood test reflect severity of an allergy?
The higher the test result, the more likely the food is actually a problem. Different factors relate to severity. The allergy test does not know if you have asthma, how much of the food you might have eaten, or your state of health at the time of an allergic reaction. The test does not know how your cells might react. The standard tests are evaluating the immune response to a selection of proteins in the food, and some of those proteins are more potent than others in some foods. Therefore, the standard tests may not reflect allergic responses to allergens within a food that causes more severe reactions. Newer tests are trying to overcome this problem (see "Delving Deeper" at the end of this chapter).

What are the advantages of a blood test over a skin test?
The blood test is not affected by your taking antihistamines, does not require rash-free areas of skin for testing, and can easily be compared from time to time as long as the same manufacturer is used.

What are the advantages of a skin test over a blood test?
The skin test gives an immediate result, can be performed with fresh or whole foods if necessary, and is much less costly than the blood test.

If the tests are not perfect, why are they done at all?
They help to provide additional evidence for or against an allergy.

Does having had a recent allergic reaction affect the test results?
There is a theoretical concern that having had a recent severe reaction might "use up" a lot of the IgE antibodies being tested, resulting in a lower or a negative test result. In practicality, we do not usually see this, but an allergist would retest in a few weeks if the test results were suspiciously negative after a severe reaction.

Can both the skin test and blood tests be negative even when there is an allergy?

Yes. This can happen if the illness is not associated with having IgE antibodies to the food (non-IgE–mediated, or cell-mediated, reactions as described in chapter 1) or because the tests did not have the right proteins.

Can you give an example of how the tests might not have the right proteins?

Sesame allergy is an example. Some of the proteins that cause allergic reactions to sesame are oil based. The skin and blood tests, however, are made from the water-based proteins. It is difficult to make tests from oil-based proteins. Therefore, if a person has a convincing allergic reaction to sesame, but the tests are negative, I remain suspicious and may try to test with the oil from sesame.

If the blood test results rise or fall over time, what does that mean?

Test results going down with time may indicate that an allergy is resolving. Results going up may indicate that the allergy is persisting. Sometimes, the test stays the same even though the person is resolving the allergy. Because high or low results reflect the chance of a true allergy, not the severity, what the result is at any point in time is as important as whether it is getting stronger or weaker.

ELIMINATION DIETS

What is an elimination diet?

An elimination diet is a prescribed diet that removes one or more suspected foods from what a person eats to determine if the food or foods are contributing to an illness.

What illnesses might be tested with an elimination diet?

Any illness that could be attributed to foods, whether the problem is allergy or any other adverse effect, could be evaluated. Typical allergic diseases that might be addressed are atopic dermatitis and chronic gastrointestinal symptoms. Elimination diets might also be used to evaluate links between foods and problems that are not considered food allergy symptoms, such as headaches, behavior, and fatigue.

Can a mother undertake an elimination diet to test her breast-fed infant?
Yes, but this must be done with careful attention to the mother's nutrition. In this situation, the mother might avoid eggs or milk, for example, to see if her infant's atopic dermatitis (allergic eczema) improves.

How long does one do an elimination diet?
Typically from a week to several weeks, which is the time frame in which chronic symptoms would be expected to resolve if the appropriate trigger were removed from the diet.

Can an elimination diet be dangerous or cause allergic problems?
Yes, in an unusual way. When a food that might be causing a chronic allergic symptom when eaten consistently is removed for an extended period (weeks or months), reintroduction might trigger a sudden and sometimes severe allergic reaction. This was first noted among children suffering from atopic dermatitis who had foods to which they tested positive removed from their diets. When they retried the food, usually months later, some experienced anaphylaxis.

Why would avoiding a tolerated food sometimes lead to becoming allergic to it?
We think the immune system may maintain a balance, with mild symptoms, while the food is eaten regularly but becomes hyper-reactive during a period of no exposure. This is an uncommon risk, but it must be considered when foods to which there is a positive test are removed from the diet for extended periods.

Can elimination diets carry nutritional consequences?
Usually, elimination diets are brief, so nutritional deficits are uncommon. However, if many foods are eliminated for long periods, working with a dietitian to assure nutritional adequacy may be required.

How does one decide what foods to eliminate in an elimination diet?

The foods are typically selected based on personal medical history, clues from epidemiologic studies showing common triggers, and test results.

What is an example of an elimination diet?

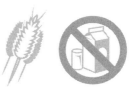

The allergist might devise a diet that avoids all major allergens and thus excludes milk, eggs, wheat, soy, peanuts, tree nuts, fish, and shellfish. Or, the doctor might prescribe a diet that has specified low-risk foods, such as a diet of chicken, rice, sweet potatoes, corn, apples, broccoli, string beans, and a calcium-fortified hypoallergenic drink.

What are the pitfalls of elimination diets for food allergy diagnosis?

One pitfall of the elimination diet is that the actual trigger may be left in the diet. Additionally, some chronic diseases have natural ups and downs in symptoms, so it may be confusing to determine if the new elimination diet is responsible for symptom improvement. Finally, elimination diets are hard, and people may be apt to see improvement for all their hard work when the underlying problem is not really different, a placebo effect.

How are individual foods identified as problematic in elimination diets?

If symptoms improve after several foods are removed, it would be unclear which of the foods was responsible. Removing one at a time, although more time consuming, would more likely identify an individual trigger. Another means to identify a specific food trigger is to add one food back at a time after symptoms have resolved to see if symptoms return. This is called an oral food challenge, or a feeding test. The oral food challenge is more definitive and can be used to address the placebo effect described above.

What is an elemental diet?

An elemental diet is one in which nutrition is provided solely by a formula that contains no whole protein, called an amino acid–based formula. In this diet, nothing being ingested could be an allergen.

Why would an elemental diet be prescribed?

This extreme diet is a definitive way to know if food is contributing to chronic symptoms. If the symptoms continue on an elemental diet, then food is not a cause.

What are the pitfalls of an elemental diet for food allergy diagnosis?

The elemental diet is extremely difficult to maintain unless it is being undertaken in an infant. People do not manage well taking no foods. Additionally, amino acid–based formulas do not taste good, although there are various flavors. Sometimes this diet is given by a feeding tube. Otherwise, pitfalls include some of the same ones that affect elimination diets, described previously. The elemental diet, however, is not plagued by the possibility that an allergen was left in the diet.

ORAL FOOD CHALLENGES (FEEDING TESTS)

What is a food challenge or feeding test?

This is a test in which a food is eaten in gradually increasing amounts under medical supervision to monitor for any symptoms, usually after the food as been eliminated from the diet for a period. The test is usually referred to as an oral food challenge.

Who does a food challenge?

Typically, an allergist suggests and supervises it.

Why is a food challenge done?

To determine if an allergy exists or has resolved. The test is not usually undertaken just to see how severe an allergy may be. The goal of a food challenge is being able to add the food back to the diet to be enjoyed frequently.

Which types of food allergies can be tested with an oral food challenge?

Any food and any type of allergy can be tested.

Can a food challenge be used to evaluate reactions to foods that are not allergic, such as behavior problems or headaches?

Yes, the oral food challenge is a "real world" test that can be used to evaluate the relationship of foods to any symptoms, even those not attributed to allergy, such as behavior problems, fatigue, or headaches. The test might be designed differently depending on the circumstances being evaluated. If you believe that eating a food for several days causes headaches or hyperactivity, then the test would be designed to mimic this situation.

How does the doctor decide if a food challenge is needed?

If the medical history and the test results are insufficient to confirm an allergy, the oral food challenge can be offered to make a definitive diagnosis.

What is an example of a situation that warrants a food challenge?

Let's say a child had a reaction to eggs three years ago, and at the time, the skin test was 5 millimeters, and the blood test was 10 kIU/L. Now the skin test is 3 millimeters, and the blood test is 2 kIU/L. These tests roughly indicate a 50% risk of her still being allergic. A feeding test would be needed to see if the allergy has resolved.

What is an example of a situation that would not warrant a food challenge?

If a child had an egg skin test of 3 millimeters and an egg IgE blood test of 2 kIU/L, the tests themselves would indicate about a 50% risk of egg allergy. If she had hives from eating eggs last week, however, a feeding test would be unnecessary because her recent reaction is confirmed to have been an egg allergy by these test results.

What factors do I need to consider in deciding if a food challenge should be done?

The allergist should discuss the chance that the food will be tolerated as well as the risks and benefits of the test. Medical history, knowledge about the food allergy, and test results are used to assess the chance that the food will be tolerated and whether the reaction might be severe if the food is not. The benefit of the challenge is no longer needing to avoid the food if it is tolerated or learning that avoidance is still needed if a reaction occurs.

Personal considerations include the importance of the food nutritionally and socially as well as the person's motivation to add the food. There are also emotional considerations for some people, such as anxiety in undergoing the test and the impact of a reaction on emotional well-being.

Can I do a food challenge at home?

Usually not, unless the allergist is certain that a trial would not result in anaphylaxis. For example, a food challenge to determine if anaphylactic allergy to peanuts has resolved would not be undertaken at home. If the problem being evaluated is whether food dyes are causing hyperactivity, however, the feedings would more likely be undertaken for longer periods at home.

How many foods can be tested at one time during a food challenge?

Usually only a single food. Sometimes an allergist may offer to test two or more foods at the same time, for example, several types of beans. The benefit of trying several foods at once is efficiency, but if a reaction occurs, one may not know which food was responsible.

How are the foods given during a food challenge?

For evaluation of allergy, the food is given in gradually increasing amounts, usually in 10- to 15-minute intervals over about 60 to 90 minutes, aiming toward a meal-sized portion. However, your allergist may alter the dosing time or amounts.

What happens if a food challenge causes an allergic reaction?

The feeding is stopped and medications are given if needed.

When does the doctor stop giving portions of the food during a food challenge?

The allergist may halt the feeding temporarily if suspicious that a reaction is starting, or permanently if a reaction is definitely occurring.

What symptoms is the doctor looking for?

Any symptoms of an allergic reaction. Some are subtle and may raise suspicion but not be clear enough to confirm that a reaction is happening. For example, complaints of mild stomachache or odd tastes in the mouth may be normal or anxiety. More obvious symptoms are hives. The allergist considers any symptoms in judging if a reaction is occurring.

Can a food challenge cause a severe allergic reaction, such as anaphylaxis?
Yes, but giving the food gradually and stopping at signs of a clear allergic reaction typically avoids severe symptoms. The purpose of this test is not to cause a severe allergic reaction but to determine if the food is tolerated. It is important that the person being tested communicate any discomfort, such as stomach pain, so that dosing can be adjusted if needed, perhaps by slowing down to see if symptoms stop or progress.

How often does a reaction occur from a food challenge?
This varies greatly and depends on the risk assessment. Most allergists will see reaction rates of less than 30% to 50%.

How often is a severe reaction triggered by a food challenge test?
Although a food challenge can cause anaphylaxis, this happens infrequently. Most reactions will need treatment only with antihistamines. Severe reactions are uncommon because the food is given gradually and feeding is stopped when symptoms begin. However, the allergist performing the test must always be prepared to treat anaphylaxis. Thankfully, no deaths from appropriately supervised oral food challenge tests have been reported that I am aware of.

How much food is given during a food challenge?
The usual goal is a meal-sized portion of the food, prepared in the manner in which it will typically be consumed.

Can a food challenge be completed without symptoms but the person be allergic anyway?
Yes. From 1% to 3% of the time, a successful oral food challenge is followed by symptoms hours later or when the food is tried again days later. These later symptoms are unlikely to be severe. It is extremely unusual,

however, for the food to cause symptoms after it has been incorporated into the diet successfully.

Can a person have symptoms during a food challenge but not be allergic?

Yes. This can happen in two main ways. Sometimes, a symptom coincidentally occurs during a food challenge. This results in falsely attributing the symptom to the food. Unfortunately, another common problem is that anxiety can result in symptoms that mimic an allergic reaction.

How can food challenges be performed with less risk of anxiety-caused false reactions?

First, you should talk to your allergist about any fears. A simple discussion can allay many of your concerns. The test itself can also be arranged in a way that reduces the chance that anxiety will affect the results. By hiding the test food in a way that masks the taste, and including placebo foods that do not contain the tested allergen but look, smell, and taste the same, it is easier to avoid false conclusions. The best way to accomplish this is a double-blind, placebo-controlled oral food challenge.

What is involved with a double-blind, placebo-controlled oral food challenge?

In this test, the food is prepared by a third party. The test food is hidden in other foods to mask the taste, and a similar tasting meal without the allergen is prepared as a placebo. The two meals are otherwise indistinguishable. They are fed in a random order under medical supervision, with neither the medical personnel nor the person being tested knowing which is which. This provides an unbiased setting for everyone involved. After the test is completed, the meal with the allergen is revealed. For example, egg powder may be hidden in one hamburger and not the other. In the morning, one hamburger is gradually eaten, and in the afternoon the other is ingested. Symptoms are recorded at each feeding and compared. If successful, these feedings are followed by eating the food in its usual form, such as scrambled eggs in this example.

What do I need to do to prepare for a food challenge?

Food challenges are usually undertaken on an empty stomach at a time when you are generally healthy. It is possible to have a very light meal if there is going to be a delay. Antihistamines should not be used prior to the test for the number of days necessary for their effect to be lost, which varies according to the type of antihistamine. Other allergy and asthma medications can be continued. The testing cannot be performed if asthma or eczema flare up on the day of scheduled testing, so these should be kept under control. Talk to your doctor if you have ongoing symptoms that might interfere with the food challenge. Be sure to discuss the risks and benefits of the tests with your allergist. You should also bring your emergency medications with you for the food challenge. Your doctor will have the medications available, but this way you will have treatments in the unlikely event that symptoms occur after you have left the office or hospital.

How can children prepare for a food challenge?

Explain to children that they might not be allergic to the food and that this test is necessary to find out if they can eat it. Explain that they might experience an allergic reaction, but if they do, the symptoms are usually mild and will be treated with medications. Let children know that this is an exception to the usual rule, that it is okay for them to try the food to which they may be allergic. Consider bringing toys, games, and appropriate distractions. Discuss with your doctor whether you should bring foods that the child enjoys that contain the allergen. Consider bringing favorite utensils and dishes to provide familiarity.

How long should one wait before having another food challenge to the same food if it was not tolerated the first time?

This depends on the food, the test results, the features of the reaction, personal preferences, and other factors. Typically, allergists wait at least a year between challenges to the same food.

What happens if the test causes an allergic reaction?

You will be instructed to continue avoiding the food. This is a disappointing outcome, but many people take comfort in having a confirmed reason to continue avoiding the food, rather than just an assumption that they have an allergy. Sometimes people also learn about the amount of food that triggers a reaction and the kinds of symptoms to expect, which can be helpful for practical reasons in daily living. For example, there may be less anxiety about trace amounts of exposure if an entire serving caused only a mild symptom.

Can an allergic reaction during a food challenge make the allergy worse or last longer?

Probably not, although this has not been studied extensively. In surveys of my patients undergoing food challenges, we did not see significant "boosting" of allergy test results after the failed food challenge. When we did see an increase, it seemed to go back down with time. Additionally, there are those who almost pass the feeding test and then pass the test the next year.

What happens if the test reveals that the food is tolerated?

In this case, the food should be added back as a regular part of the diet. Let your doctor know if you have any suspicion that the food is causing a problem. Be careful to avoid other foods you are allergic to when purchasing new foods that contain the now acceptable ingredient.

Can a food allergy return after a successful food challenge?

It is possible to develop an allergy to any food at any age, so having a recurrence of an allergy is a theoretical possibility. Recurrence of an allergy after successfully passing an oral food challenge, however, is very uncommon. It has happened with peanut allergies, but almost all individuals who reported recurrence after a successful challenge had not incorporated peanuts into their diets. Their symptoms occurred when they tried peanuts again about a year following the successful food challenge. In contrast, it appears that those who did incorporate peanuts into their diets did not experience these problems. This is why it is suggested to eat the food regularly after a successful ingestion test.

How often does the food have to be eaten after a successfully passed oral food challenge?

There is no specific regimen for incorporating the food. Including it in the diet should not be stressful. Simply ingest the food periodically, as one would do naturally, and don't avoid it any longer.

What are the possible emotional consequences of a food challenge test?
You would probably think that a "failed" test would lead to sadness and increased anxiety, but studies have actually shown that a failed test can often improve quality of life. When people know that they are avoiding a food for a good reason and have faced the potential unknown of what a reaction is like, they often feel empowered. Everyone is different, however, and you should discuss how a "failed" feeding test might affect you or your child. Sometimes professional mental health counseling is needed before or after a food challenge to reduce anxiety.

ADDITIONAL TESTS

What other tests might be done for food allergy?
Additional tests that are not routinely performed include patch testing, basophil activation testing, component testing, and total IgE. There are also several tests that are not recommended or are considered unproved.

What is a food patch test?
This test is performed by placing the food on the skin, usually under a small metal cap, for a day or two. Two or three days after removal, the area is checked for rash.

Why would a food patch test be performed?
This test has been used to evaluate illnesses that might not produce immediate allergic reactions as well as illnesses in which IgE antibodies to the food are not produced. These conditions include eosinophilic esophagitis, food protein–induced enterocolitis syndrome, and atopic dermatitis (eczema). The theory is that these delayed allergic reactions on the skin patch test may reflect the chronic or delayed reactions of these illnesses.

Is the food patch test painful?
No, but it can be itchy and uncomfortable. It is sometimes difficult to keep a test in place because of irritation and sweating.

Can a food patch test cause a severe reaction?
Having a food touch the skin is not likely to result in severe reactions.

Is the food patch test accurate?
The accuracy of the test has not been confirmed, and it is not a widely accepted procedure. It is still being studied.

Is the food patch test a routinely performed food allergy test?
No. It is not studied well enough to be considered a standard or routine allergy test.

What is a basophil activation test?
A basophil activation test is a laboratory test in which a food is mixed with allergy cells to see if the cells respond. This is quite similar to a skin test except that it is performed in a test tube. This test shows some promise but is still not routinely performed.

What is a test for total IgE?
A test for total IgE measures all IgE antibodies in the bloodstream. Total IgE does not give any specific diagnostic information. Sometimes allergists perform this test to get a relative idea of the proportion of food-specific IgE, but studies have so far not shown that determining total IgE reliably assists in diagnosing a specific food allergy.

What is an intradermal test?
An intradermal test is a skin test that is performed by injecting a small amount of extract into the skin, rather than simply scratching or pricking it. This method is not recommended because it is too likely to result in positive results that are meaningless (false positive) and it carries the risk of causing a generalized allergic reaction.

What is component testing?

A food is made up of many different proteins that may have varying effects on allergy outcomes. Component testing separates the different proteins in a single food and measures IgE against the separate proteins. This type of testing holds promise for improved accuracy over current tests. Although component testing has not yet been validated well enough for widespread use, allergists are using it to gain insights in specific situations. See more in the "Delving Deeper" section of this chapter.

UNPROVEN AND DISPROVEN TESTS

What tests are not considered helpful?

Several tests are considered unproven and are not recommended by food allergy experts. These include applied kinesiology, provocation-neutralization, resistance testing, cytotoxic testing, and IgG / IgG4 testing.

What is applied kinesiology?

An applied kinesiology test has the individual hold a food, often in a glass bottle, while muscle strength is being checked, with a notion that weakness indicates an allergy. There is no clear scientific basis for the test. When the approach was subject to blinding (hiding the bottle contents from the practitioner), the results varied, indicating that some degree of suggestion or bias is likely at work when this testing is performed.

What is provocation-neutralization?

The food is given in small amounts (doses) that increase until symptoms are provoked (provocation), and then a lower dose is given to stop the symptoms (neutralization). This is usually done by mouth, but sometimes by injection. The symptoms tested are usually subjective (fatigue, drowsiness, skin itch, pain, chills, stomach upset, and so forth) and not typical of allergies. About fifteen studies looked at the effectiveness of this approach, but only eight were done without the provider knowing the doses and substances, and only one was done with a comparison group. Several of the studies showed poor results, including a 70% rate of improvement using false treatments. In one widely publicized study that was properly performed, with the testing blinded and a comparison group included, provocation-neutralization was not effective (using salt water had the same result as using the treatment extracts). It seems that the approach relies on the placebo effect and the suggestion of improvement from the person doing the test.

What is VEGA, or resistance testing?

Electronic equipment measures the flow of electricity through the body with the idea that variations indicate a potential allergy. The person being tested holds the food in hand or on an aluminum plate. Sometimes the testing is done for a child by testing the parent, who holds the child's hand. Readouts and printouts are made by a computer. A controlled study shows no difference in results between people with or without allergies. There is no reason to expect this test to be useful and no proof that it is helpful. There are additional electronic systems claiming, for example, to use laser technology, which remain unproved.

What is IgG / IgG4 testing?

IgG, or IgG4, are antibodies (proteins) that can recognize food proteins. Although tests are sold to measure these antibodies, having them does not appear to correlate with specific allergies. In fact, in studies attempting to treat food allergies, these antibodies appear to increase when the treatment is going well. Additionally, individuals who do not react to foods have these antibodies. Therefore, these tests are not recommended to diagnose a food allergy. Their role in monitoring resolution of food allergies is under study.

What is hair analysis?

Hair is analyzed to somehow determine allergies. Laboratories claiming to be able to diagnose allergies this way were put to the test decades ago and failed. Body chemical analysis is a related test, where blood or other body fluids are tested for various chemicals. Anyone can have these various chemicals in their bodies, and a relation to allergy is not known or proved.

What is a pulse test?

Checking the pulse as a way to measure response to a food was suggested in the 1940s. One might guess that the pulse would change during a severe allergic reaction, but the test has no dependable diagnostic value.

What are cytotoxic testing and ALCAT?

Both tests measure cell responses to foods. Cytotoxic testing looks at cell death under a microscope, and the ALCAT test measures the size of cells as a reflection of their activity. There is no strong scientific rationale behind these tests nor large-scale studies supporting their use.

Why do people do tests that traditional allergists and expert panels recommend against?

These tests have failed to pass scientific rigor, but they are not outlawed. Unfortunately, "buyer beware" is the current situation with allergy testing.

Delving Deeper:
IMPROVED DIAGNOSTIC TESTS AND COMPONENT TESTING

What is on the horizon for improved diagnostic tests?

The goal of improved food allergy diagnostic testing is to have tests that are able to predict allergies more accurately and provide insights into severity and prognosis.

How does component testing work?

Recall that every food is a collection of proteins, and each protein may differ in being a potent or less potent allergen. Component testing separately measures IgE responses to the various proteins in a single food rather than as a mixture. For example, peanuts would no longer be thought of as one item to be tested, but would be approached as a collection of proteins, with allergic responses to each individual protein having potential meaning. A person whose immune system recognizes (creates antibodies against) only the peanut proteins that are easily digested may be less likely to have a severe reaction than a person whose system recognizes proteins that are resistant to digestion and more likely to enter the bloodstream.

A specific example is a peanut protein called Ara h 2. This protein is resistant to digestion and is associated with severe reactions. In contrast, a protein called Ara h 8 is digested easily. If the component testing is negative to Ara h 2 (the more potent allergen) and only positive to Ara h 8 (the weaker allergen), there may be no peanut allergy or only a mild one. Tests like this are already on the market for many foods, including eggs, milk, wheat, soy, peanuts, tree nuts, fruits, and vegetables.

Component tests are being used increasingly by allergists to give additional insights into the nature of an individual's food allergy, sometimes helping to decide, for example, if it is reasonable to perform a physician-supervised feeding test. However, further study is needed to be able to use this test more accurately. As with the standard tests, the degree of immune response (for example, how much IgE is detecting the protein) to each "component" may be informative to determine allergy risks, and this has only begun to be studied. However, the approach holds great promise for improved diagnosis. The tests are increasingly being studied and increasingly being approved as valid tests.

What is epitope testing?

Every food protein has various areas on it that the immune system might recognize. The exact areas recognized may reflect different risks of having an allergic response. For example, a child making IgE antibodies to segments of a single milk protein that survives digestion may be less likely to outgrow milk allergy and be prone to more severe reactions than a child whose IgE antibodies recognize only segments of milk protein that do not survive digestion. Studies have been promising. These tests are undergoing additional research to see if they can be commercialized.

What is affinity testing?

The strength with which the IgE attaches to protein, its "affinity," may influence the severity or persistence of an allergy. The stronger the attachment, the more likely the allergy will be severe or persistent. More studies are needed to investigate this possibility, but early studies have shown promise in using this approach to distinguish children with transient or persistent milk allergy.

Also of Interest:
REASONS FOR UNEXPECTED TEST RESULTS

Why would a test be positive if the person can eat the food?

One explanation has to do with digestion. When the food is placed on the skin for testing, it is not digested. There may be IgE antibodies that recognize the undigested protein, leading to the skin response—a positive test. After the food is eaten, the proteins become digested and may not be recognized by those same IgE antibodies. Therefore, the skin test is positive, but the food is tolerated when eaten. Another explanation has to do with the amount of IgE antibodies. There may be enough to cause a skin response or be detected in a blood test but not enough to activate enough allergy cells to cause symptoms when the food is eaten.

Why do allergy test results go up or down when the food is not being eaten?

We do not know why test results rise, fall, or stay the same. When a test shows increase, it usually means the allergy is not waning. Whether the food was eaten does not appear to relate to this rise. One explanation could be that the body's total production of IgE is increasing, so the antibodies to the food being tested are simply rising along with it (similar to a child growing). Perhaps the food being tested has proteins similar to those in pollens and the person has developed new or stronger pollen allergies. Maybe there are exposures to the food that are not triggering reactions beyond heightening the immune response. On the other hand, we know that at least for some people, exposures do not result in increases in the test result. In summary, an increase in a test result may not be traceable to a lack of strict avoidance of the food.

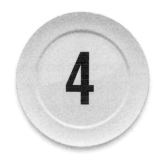

What Is **ANAPHYLAXIS** and How Do I Treat It?

In this chapter I answer questions about how to recognize and treat anaphylaxis, a severe allergic reaction. Understanding the symptoms and treatments is essential to protect yourself and others from the most dangerous type of food allergy reaction.

GENERAL QUESTIONS ON ANAPHYLAXIS

What is anaphylaxis?

Anaphylaxis is a severe allergic reaction that is rapid in onset and can be fatal. Symptoms occur beyond where the food has made contact, beyond the mouth and gut. Typically, several areas of the body are affected, for example, the skin and the gut, or the gut and breathing.

What is anaphylactic shock?

When anaphylaxis leads to poor blood circulation that deprives the body of oxygen and nutrients, it is called "shock."

What foods cause anaphylaxis?

Any food can potentially cause anaphylaxis, but the ones that do so most often are peanuts, tree nuts, shellfish, fish, milk, and eggs.

Who is at risk of anaphylaxis?

Anyone could develop a food allergy that results in anaphylaxis. The risks of food anaphylaxis are the same as those for food allergy: having a family or personal history of allergic problems, such as asthma, atopic dermatitis (eczema), hay fever, or food allergies. Allergies to foods that more often cause severe reactions, namely peanuts, tree nuts, fish, and shellfish, may represent an increased risk. Persons with co-existing asthma appear to have a higher risk of more severe food-allergic reactions.

What are the symptoms of anaphylaxis?

No specific symptom defines anaphylaxis. Symptoms might occur in any of several body areas (systems) and may involve various symptoms in each of them.

- Skin: hives, itchy rashes, swelling (such as of the eyes or lips)
- Breathing: shortness of breath, wheezing, chest tightness, repetitive coughing, throat tightness, hoarseness, trouble breathing or swallowing, drooling, obstructive swelling of the tongue
- Gut: vomiting, cramping pain, diarrhea
- Circulation: pale or blue skin, faintness, weak pulse, dizziness, confusion
- Other symptoms: feeling of "impending doom," odd tastes in the mouth, uterine contractions

How long after eating a food can anaphylaxis happen?

From minutes to about two hours. It is rare for symptoms to begin more than two hours after the food was eaten, and unusual for them to begin more than an hour afterward. Some symptoms will usually begin within 20 minutes.

What pattern of symptoms would definitely be anaphylaxis?

There is no single pattern. A few hives or isolated gut symptoms would not qualify as anaphylaxis, but combinations of symptoms would. Therefore, a person with hives and vomiting from a food-allergic reaction is experiencing anaphylaxis. A severe symptom after a food is eaten could qualify as anaphylaxis even if it is the only symptom. For example, a person with poor blood circulation after ingesting a food allergen is experiencing anaphylaxis.

If there are no hives, can one assume anaphylaxis is not occurring?
No. It is possible to have anaphylaxis without any skin symptoms. Knowing this is VERY important because fatalities have been attributed to ignoring treatment of anaphylaxis for lack of seeing a rash.

Are there specific symptoms during anaphylaxis that are dangerous?
Yes.

What are the most serious symptoms during anaphylaxis?
Any symptoms affecting breathing or circulation are serious. Breathing symptoms include shortness of breath, wheezing, chest tightness, repetitive coughing, throat tightness, hoarseness, trouble breathing or swallowing, drooling, and obstructive swelling of the tongue. Blood circulation symptoms include pale or blue skin, confusion, and passing out. A feeling of "impending doom" can also precede serious symptoms.

What are the milder symptoms during anaphylaxis?
Skin rashes and swelling, mouth itch, and gut symptoms are not intrinsically dangerous.

Besides foods, what else triggers anaphylaxis?
Triggers include medications, insect stings, vaccinations, latex, and anaphylaxis for no clear reason, called idiopathic anaphylaxis.

Are there illnesses that mimic anaphylaxis?
There are several. Among them are scombroid fish poisoning (spoilage of dark-meat fish that releases histamine-like toxins), panic attacks, choking, heart attacks, and allergic responses such as asthma or hives.

How can one tell an asthma exacerbation from anaphylaxis?

It may be tricky. Asthma triggers include viral infections, exercise, cold air, and inhalation of allergens, such as pollens or animal dander. Isolated wheezing after these triggers is most likely asthma. Asthma symptoms of cough and wheeze without other symptoms, such as itchy mouth or hives, and without a known or likely exposure to a food allergen are most likely due to an asthma flare.

What should you do if you are not sure a reaction is truly anaphylaxis or another medical problem?

If there is a suspicion of anaphylaxis, it is best to treat a person for it. In all cases, administer first-aid management and activate emergency health care responses, for example, by calling 911.

How long does anaphylaxis last?

In most cases, the anaphylactic reaction lasts under an hour when treated appropriately. Sometimes symptoms return over the subsequent hours. Rarely, anaphylaxis symptoms can continue in waves for days.

How often does anaphylaxis have more than one wave of symptoms?

It depends on the severity of the first wave of symptoms. If the first wave was mild, a second wave is less likely to occur. Studies have estimated that the second wave occurs in 1% to 20% of reactions. Sometimes the second wave is more severe.

What is the timing of additional waves of symptoms during anaphylaxis?

If additional waves of symptoms occur at all, they usually happen within a few hours of the onset of the reaction. It is therefore recommended to stay under medical supervision for at least four hours after a reaction has subsided. This instruction would vary based on the severity of the reaction—longer if serious symptoms occurred.

How quickly can an allergic reaction progress from mild to severe?

Within minutes. However, progression of symptoms can also occur over hours.

How do I know when anaphylaxis is going to happen?
Unfortunately, it is not predictable.

Why do I need to understand how to recognize anaphylaxis?
Because prompt treatment is needed to address the symptoms adequately.

How often is anaphylaxis fatal?
Rarely, but the risk is greater if treatment is delayed.

What are the risks for fatal food anaphylaxis?
Studies of people who experienced fatal allergic reactions revealed the main factors they seemed to share and the presumed reasons these factors are risks. The risk factors for fatal reactions include

- Delayed treatment with epinephrine

- Being a teenager / young adult

- Having asthma

- Having a diagnosed food allergy

- Having a history of reactions to trace exposures

- Having the reaction away from home

- Not having hives during the fatal episode

- Being allergic to peanuts, tree nuts, fish, shellfish, or milk

Why is delayed treatment with epinephrine a risk for fatal food anaphylaxis?
Epinephrine is the primary treatment for anaphylaxis. Waiting too long may make treatment less effective. In one study of children and teens with severe food-allergic reactions, the ones who survived received epinephrine by about 15 minutes after symptoms began whereas those who died did not receive treatment until about an hour after symptoms began.

Why are teenagers and young adults at greater risk for fatal food anaphylaxis?
Presumably these are individuals who are more likely to eat risky foods and not treat their symptoms promptly.

Why is having co-existing asthma a risk for fatal food anaphylaxis?

It is believed that having asthma, or "twitchy airways," makes the airways more vulnerable to becoming reactive during a food-allergic reaction. Therefore, a person with asthma who experiences an allergic reaction to a food is more likely to have breathing difficulties during the reaction, which is a severe symptom.

Why is having a previously diagnosed food allergy a risk for fatal food anaphylaxis?

We do not know exactly. Although a first allergic reaction is occasionally fatal, most who have succumbed had a known allergy.

Why is having a history of reactions to trace exposures a risk for fatal food anaphylaxis?

Those who are more sensitive may be at higher risk.

Why is having a reaction away from home a risk for fatal food anaphylaxis?

Presumably, being in unfamiliar settings or not having access to medications can be a risk, which is why education about avoidance and always having a prescribed treatment available is so important.

Why is a lack of hives during anaphylaxis associated with fatal outcomes?

Presumably, there is an erroneous assumption that anaphylaxis must include hives. This assumption may lead to delayed treatment if symptoms do not include hives. The lesson is, anaphylaxis can occur without hives.

Why are anaphylactic reactions to peanuts, tree nuts, fish, shellfish, and milk associated with fatal outcomes?

These are the foods most often associated with severe reactions, although any food can trigger anaphylaxis. Peanuts and tree nuts account for the majority of fatal reactions.

How does one prevent fatal anaphylaxis?

Avoiding the trigger and seeking prompt treatment are the only current preventive treatments.

What should be done for a person having anaphylaxis?
Prompt treatment with epinephrine and alerting emergency medical care, for example, by calling 911.

When calling 911 about food anaphylaxis, what should they be told?
They should be told that the person is experiencing anaphylaxis, whatever treatments were given, and how they are doing. Some states do not automatically have treatments for allergy available on an ambulance, so explaining the situation may ensure that they dispatch the correct emergency unit, one that has medications such as epinephrine.

Why go to an emergency room for anaphylaxis?
A person who is experiencing or has recently experienced anaphylaxis should be taken to an emergency room for evaluation and possibly additional treatments that are available there. An emergency room is preferable to a doctor's office because the office is less likely to be well equipped to treat a progressive reaction.

How long should a person who experienced anaphylaxis stay in an emergency room?
Generally, at least four hours to be observed for recurrence of symptoms. The observation period might be longer if the symptoms were severe or continued to occur.

My doctor told me to always go to an emergency room if I inject epinephrine. Why?
Many people erroneously think that injecting epinephrine is itself the reason to go to an emergency room, as if the epinephrine might cause a medical problem. This MISCONCEPTION can lead to a person being reluctant to inject the epinephrine. The reason you should go to an emergency room afterward is that you experienced a serious allergic reaction that needs to be monitored in case symptoms worsen or recur.

What plans should be in place for a person at risk of anaphylaxis?
A person who is at risk for food anaphylaxis should be prescribed

self-injectable epinephrine, be trained in how and when to use it, and be educated about allergen avoidance.

Are there any situations that increase a person's risk for food anaphylaxis?
For a person with a food allergy, several circumstances might increase the risk of a more severe or anaphylactic allergic reaction, including eating a larger amount of the food, exercise, taking aspirin or alcohol, and having co-existing asthma.

What is the relationship between exercise, food, and anaphylaxis?
Some people can eat a specific food or foods and have no symptoms unless they exercise near the time of the meal. This problem is called food-associated exercise-induced anaphylaxis (FAEIA). Sometimes any food will cause this problem, but more often specific ones do. The most common triggers are wheat, celery, and seafood. Treatment requires avoidance of the food for at least four hours prior to exercise. A person with FAEIA should always exercise with a buddy and have anaphylaxis treatments on hand.

In addition, eating a food to which you are allergic and then exercising may increase the severity of a reaction.

How do aspirin or alcohol increase the risk of food anaphylaxis?
Most likely by making the stomach lining more prone to quickly absorb food allergens into the bloodstream.

How does asthma increase the risk of anaphylaxis?
If the lungs are already vulnerable to asthma, an allergic reaction to foods might more likely result in breathing symptoms, making the reaction more severe.

What can be done to improve safety for teenagers at risk for anaphylaxis?
We think that teenagers are a high-risk group because they are more likely to eat a food without making sure it is safe and are less likely to promptly treat a reaction. Our studies suggest that social reasons (peer pressure, feeling different) and possibly a teenager's feeling of invincibility are the

main factors. When we asked teens about their allergies, they indicated that they wanted others to better understand food allergies. They were less likely to carry medications when they assumed there was less risk (sports, dance without foods) or did not have a convenient means to carry them. Based on these studies, I think it is essential for readers (especially parents, teachers, coaches, and so forth) to address the following problems related to teenagers with food allergies:

Problem: Misperception of "anaphylaxis"

- Teach the symptoms to look out for, not just the word "anaphylaxis"

Problem: Low rate of autoinjector use

- Educate about treatment circumstances (the need to inject promptly, when to inject)
- Review injector technique
- Work with your doctor to make sure the teenager is comfortable and confident in using the medication

Problem: Inconsistency in carrying autoinjector, varying by social circumstances (less at parties), perceived risks (less at sporting activities), and convenience (clothing that does not have pockets)

- Impress on the teenager the need for consistency
- Issue reminders to carry consistently, especially to sport and social activities
- Offer alternatives that make carrying the autoinjector easier (purse, holster)
- Have an autoinjector on-site when appropriate (for example, coaches, teachers)

Problem: Risky eating

- Review risks of exposures and discourage risky behavior

- Supervise early practice in obtaining safe foods, to instill good habits

- Encourage peer education

Problem: Feeling "different" or "less concerned," leading to risk taking

- Encourage third-party education about allergies, especially for friends

- Encourage peers to work together to protect the teen who has the food allergy

  – The Food Allergy & Anaphylaxis Network, now merged with the Food Allergy Initiative, has a program called PAL (Protect A Life), which encourages peer education and shared responsibilities

Problem: Difficulty in obtaining safe foods

- Increase safe food options

- Assign a "point person" for safe meals (for example, in the cafeteria)

What should I be discussing with my food-allergic teenager?

Start conversations on food allergy topics well before problems (risk taking) might arise. Ask your teen, "What would you do if you had a reaction at a party or with friends?" Discuss times when your teen might think it is not necessary to carry medications, and explore options to make consistent carrying easy to do. Discuss peer pressure. Discuss dating (and kissing). Discuss when epinephrine would be used. Openly discuss any resistance about self-injection. Discuss how to approach dining out with friends. Emphasize that alcohol use can result in increased risk taking. Emphasize that independence requires increasing acceptance of responsibility. Involve your allergist in these conversations as well.

EPINEPHRINE

What is epinephrine?

Epinephrine is a medication similar to adrenaline, which is made by the body during a "fight or flight" reaction. Epinephrine reduces swelling, opens the breathing tubes, tightens blood vessels to carry blood more effectively, and strengthens the heart beat.

What symptoms does epinephrine treat?

Epinephrine treats all the severe symptoms of anaphylaxis, reducing throat swelling and wheezing and improving blood circulation.

How is epinephrine given?

By injection.

Who should be prescribed epinephrine?

Anyone who is considered at risk for anaphylaxis.

How is it determined that a person is at risk for food anaphylaxis?

Your doctor must decide whether this is the case, but certainly epinephrine should be prescribed for anyone who has already experienced severe allergic reactions to foods. Persons considered at risk may include anyone with food allergies, but especially allergies to peanuts, tree nuts, shellfish, or fish. Prescriptions of self-injectable epinephrine are usually considered for anyone who has more than a mild type of food allergy (for example, oral allergy syndrome), especially for those who also have asthma. Some physicians prescribe it even for people with milder reactions.

Where on the body is epinephrine injected?

In the middle part of the upper leg, roughly midway between the front and side.

Can the injection be given through clothing?

Yes, although it is a good idea to take a few extra seconds to pull pants down or lift up a dress to avoid hitting a seam or something in a pocket that might block the injection.

When should epinephrine be given?

Whenever anaphylaxis is occurring or is likely to develop, epinephrine should be injected promptly. As described previously, combinations of symptoms in different areas of the body, or any severe symptoms after a known or likely food allergen was eaten, would indicate that anaphylaxis is occurring and warrant injection of epinephrine.

Why is it necessary to inject epinephrine promptly during anaphylaxis?

Getting the most benefit from epinephrine throughout the body requires adequate blood circulation to carry it. If one waits too long, the heart and circulation may not be able to get the medication where it is needed.

Should epinephrine be given before anaphylaxis if there are allergic symptoms?

There are situations when the answer is "yes." This takes some judgment, but if a person with a known severe allergy has definitely eaten an allergen, it is reasonable to inject epinephrine without waiting for symptoms that indicate anaphylaxis.

Should epinephrine ever be given before any allergic symptoms develop?

Sometimes it is a good decision to inject epinephrine even before any symptoms develop. A situation where this might be reasonable is when a person definitely ingested the food allergen that has caused extremely severe allergic reactions in the past.

What symptoms of an allergic reaction would not require epinephrine?

In general, if there are only mild symptoms, such as several hives, some stomach upset, or mouth itching, epinephrine can usually be withheld because other medications can treat the mild symptoms. There should be careful monitoring, however, to watch for any progression of symptoms that may warrant epinephrine.

How fast does epinephrine work?
Usually there is relief within minutes.

How long do the effects of epinephrine last?
The medication effects last for about 20 to 30 minutes, but usually only one dose is needed.

How often does a person need more than one dose of epinephrine?
This happens about 10% to 20% of the time.

What would be a reason to give more than one dose of epinephrine?
If the symptoms did not respond well enough or they recur, more doses can be given.

How long should you wait before giving a second dose of epinephrine?
Guidelines state 5 to 20 minutes. However, if a person is having severe trouble breathing or is not responding well because of poor blood circulation, giving another dose in less than 5 minutes may be reasonable.

How many doses of epinephrine should a food-allergic person carry?
Generally two, because a second dose might be needed.

How does an autoinjector work?
A premeasured amount of epinephrine is injected from a spring-loaded injector.

What autoinjectors of epinephrine are available?
Several different brands are on the market, with more in the pipeline to come. Some brands that have been or are scheduled to be available in the United States are EpiPen, Auvi-Q, Twinject, and Adrenaclick. Whatever device you and your doctor decide on, the crucial point to discuss is how to activate the medication. If your pharmacist dispenses a device you are not familiar with, discuss this immediately with the pharmacist and your doctor.

How many doses of epinephrine are in an autoinjector?

Most autoinjectors have one dose and are discarded after use. The Twin-ject device autoinjects a first dose and has a second dose available in the same unit, but the unit must be opened to access a syringe for the second dose, which is injected manually. If only the autoinjected dose is used, and no second dose is needed, the unit is still disposed of and not reused.

Is epinephrine always effective to treat anaphylaxis?

Epinephrine is very effective, especially when given promptly for anaphy-laxis. However, there are reports of fatal food anaphylaxis despite appro-priate treatment with epinephrine. This is why you should NEVER take risks with your diet thinking that if you have a reaction, you can simply depend on the epinephrine. One of the reported deaths was in a teenager who took risks when thinking this way.

How can I learn and teach others about how to use an epinephrine autoinjector?

You should ask your doctor to demonstrate how and when to use the device, using a trainer. You can also look at videos online from the man-ufacturer's website. If you have an expired device, you can practice by injecting into an orange. But do not eat the orange! And take the expired device to your doctor or local hospital for disposal.

What if epinephrine is given but the person was not having anaphylaxis?

Epinephrine is a safe medication, which is one reason it is better to use it if in doubt. Whether given to a person having anaphylaxis or not, the side effects are the same. This medication was routinely used to treat asthma before asthma inhalers became the main therapy.

Can repeated use of epinephrine make it less effective?

No. People do not become resistant to the effects of epinephrine from prior use.

What are the side effects of epinephrine?

The most common side effects are increased heart rate and some jitteriness or tremor, similar to having too much caffeine. A person may also develop a headache and appear pale or sometimes flushed.

Is epinephrine dangerous?

No. There is some risk for people with heart problems who may not tolerate a faster heart rate, but epinephrine should be injected for anaphylaxis even if there is a heart problem. Persons with a known heart condition should discuss their anaphylactic food allergy with their physician.

Can epinephrine be injected into a pregnant woman?

Epinephrine should be injected to treat anaphylaxis in a pregnant woman.

Are there any medications that should not be taken if epinephrine is prescribed?

Some medications, such as beta blockers, could interact poorly with the epinephrine, and alternative medications to treat heart problems or high blood pressure could be chosen. Talk to your doctor about these alternatives. Because anaphylaxis is life threatening, it is recommended to inject epinephrine for anaphylaxis even if a person has heart problems or is on medications that may interact poorly.

How long do epinephrine side effects last?

Usually for under 30 minutes.

Do autoinjectors expire?

Yes. Always check the expiration date. When new, they should be dated for at least a year. If your pharmacist gives you one with an expiration date in less than a year, ask for a newer one.

What if I forgot to replace an expired autoinjector but that is all that I have to treat anaphylaxis?

While it would be preferable to have an unexpired autoinjector, if there is anaphylaxis and no other options, an expired autoinjector is better than not using any. There is likely to be some active medication remaining.

What should I do with my expired epinephrine autoinjector?

First, make sure you have new autoinjectors available. You can use the expired ones to practice injecting into an orange, as described above. Take the used or expired autoinjector to your doctor or local emergency room to be disposed of as medical waste.

Why does the epinephrine autoinjector have a window?

If the medication went bad for some reason, it can become discolored with a brown hue. The window allows one to check if this has happened.

How do I store an epinephrine autoinjector?

The manufacturers generally suggest that it be stored at room temperature, which is generally between 68 and 77 degrees Fahrenheit (20 to 25 degrees Celsius), with allowable temperature fluctuations of 59 to 86 degrees Fahrenheit (15 to 30 degrees Celsius). This is usually achieved by carrying it on your person or in a carrying pouch. If you are going to be in extremes of heat or cold, you could store it in a cooler, a temperature-resistant pouch, or an empty Thermos. Do not leave the unit in a glove compartment in the heat or freezing cold.

If I left an autoinjector in extreme heat or cold, how do I know if it was damaged?

You may not. If the liquid in the clear window has become cloudy or brown, the injector needs to be replaced. However, exposure to extreme temperatures might compromise the injector without any obvious changes. If you suspect there was exposure to an extreme temperature, replace the injector.

How does the doctor decide on the dose of epinephrine for autoinjectors?

The unit comes as a 0.15 milligram (sometimes called a "junior") or a 0.3 milligram dose. Manufacturers generally suggest the 0.15 mg unit for those weighing between 33 and 66 pounds (15 to 30 kilograms) and the 0.3 mg unit for those at and above 66 pounds. Because under-dosing is likely for children just under 66 pounds, however, several expert groups suggest switching to the 0.3 mg dose at approximately 55 pounds (25 kilograms). Your doctor may suggest switching at slightly different weights depending on your specific history.

What can be done to give epinephrine to infants who are too small for the lowest autoinjector dose?

This is a difficult situation because the alternative to an autoinjector is to have a glass vial of epinephrine and a syringe that would need to be filled at the time of a reaction. Studies suggest that using this means of treatment can be prone to errors. Many pediatricians may be comfortable with prescribing an autoinjector for infants over 22 pounds (10 kilograms), but this is individualized according to specific medical circumstances. Because alternatives are few, your doctor may discuss having the smaller dose autoinjector available even if your infant is under 22 pounds.

Does the injection hurt?

It feels like a pinch, but people often describe the relief they feel from symptoms rather than the pain from the injection.

How can I overcome fear of self-injection?

If you think that you or your child would be reluctant to self-inject, you should discuss this openly with your physician. The safety of the medication should be emphasized, but some people have an aversion to needles that increases their reluctance to self-inject. Some allergists have advocated for having patients self-inject in the office, just to allay fear about doing it during a reaction. Another approach is to use a sterile needle and syringe, under medical supervision, with no injection of medication, just to build confidence that the self-injection can be done.

What if I injected my finger with epinephrine by accident?

This is a common error when a person is attempting to give the treatment to another person. It underscores why it is essential to review how to use the injectors and to practice with trainers. If the thumb is accidentally injected, the blood vessels in the finger may spasm, reducing blood flow. This usually resolves by itself, but if your finger is discolored, you should go to an emergency room for treatment with a paste or injection that reverses the problem. Also, don't forget to use another injector to administer the epinephrine to the person who needs it.

ANTIHISTAMINES

What does an antihistamine do?
Antihistamines block the histamine that is released from allergy cells during an allergic reaction. Histamine is partly responsible for the itching, redness, and swelling during an allergic reaction. Many powerful chemicals are released during anaphylaxis, however, and an antihistamine cannot treat anaphylaxis.

If antihistamines cannot treat anaphylaxis, why do symptoms sometimes get better with antihistamines alone?
Allergic reactions may improve on their own, or the symptoms may be mild enough to respond to the antihistamines.

What antihistamines are available?
There are many over-the-counter antihistamines, as well as a few prescription types. They can be sold under brand names or generic names. The "side," or inactive, ingredients may differ among the formulations and between the brands and the generics. Examples of popular over-the-counter antihistamines include diphenhydramine (Benadryl), cetirizine (Zyrtec), and fexofenadine (Allegra). There are various formulations (liquid, tablet, capsules, meltaways, melting strips, and so on). All antihistamines have generally the same actions, reducing itching and swelling. Their onset of action, length of action, and degree of sedation (sleepiness) can differ. The two forms used most often for food-allergic reactions are diphenhydramine and cetirizine. Watch out for combination forms (for example, those with decongestant or pain medications in the same formulation) that are sold to treat various cold and flu symptoms. For an allergic reaction, you want to purchase the basic types that have one active ingredient.

How long does it take for an antihistamine to work?

About 30 minutes for diphenhydramine and cetirizine. When symptoms appear to improve promptly after taking an antihistamine, this usually means the symptoms would have improved on their own without treatment.

Does it matter what form of antihistamine is taken (pill, liquid, dissolvable, or other form)?

For additional treatment during anaphylaxis, use a form that can be absorbed as quickly as possible. Thus, all forms *except* capsules and pills might be preferentially used. Often, convenience is an issue because the antihistamines are carried along with epinephrine in a "kit" or pack. Some people prefer to carry dissolvable forms or premeasured foil pouches. You should explore options and practice opening the different forms to see what works best for you.

How are antihistamines dosed?

The dosing of diphenhydramine is generally 12.5 milligrams for every 22 pounds, up to about 50 mg. The dosing for cetirizine is generally 2.5 mg for ages 2 through 5 and 5 to 10 mg for ages 6 and older. Your doctor may suggest slightly different dosing for use during an allergic reaction, usually going toward the higher ranges for weight or age.

Should antihistamines be part of a treatment plan for anaphylaxis?

They generally are to add additional comfort care.

What are the side effects of antihistamines?

Most forms cause sedation, but the degree of sedation can differ. For example, diphenhydramine is more sedating, in general, than cetirizine. Some people experience the opposite effect, feeling restless.

In anaphylaxis, what should be given first, epinephrine or an antihistamine?

If anaphylaxis is occurring, the priority is to give epinephrine.

If symptoms are not getting better after a dose of antihistamines, can more be given?

Many physicians might suggest taking a bit more antihistamine, but it must also be appreciated that it can take 30 minutes for the dose to take effect. The types of symptoms must be considered as well. Any progressive symptoms or severe symptoms, as described in the previous sections, should be treated with epinephrine, without waiting for or expecting the antihistamine to treat these symptoms.

If a person is already taking antihistamines for a condition like hay fever, and they have a food-allergic reaction, can more antihistamines be taken?

Yes, this is a reasonable approach.

Can being on an antihistamine for hay fever or another allergic problem reduce having early and mild symptoms after a food allergen is eaten?

Yes. For example, it may reduce mouth itch or some hives. It would not necessarily affect progression of a reaction to anaphylaxis. Again, antihistamines do not treat anaphylaxis!

Is it dangerous or problematic to be on an antihistamine continuously if you have a severe food allergy?

There is a hypothetical concern that being on an antihistamine might reduce the milder initial symptoms of an allergic reaction, resulting in the person continuing to eat a food with an allergen and perhaps getting a larger dose of the food. Allergists, however, advocate appropriate treatment of allergic conditions with antihistamines regardless of there being a potentially severe food allergy. There is no reason to suffer with hay fever or itchy skin rashes because of a theoretical concern about using antihistamines. Additionally, to maintain safety, it is not appropriate to depend on experiencing initial mild symptoms from a meal (which often does not occur even off antihistamines). One should be careful to obtain safe foods through label reading and good communication. Whether or not mild initial symptoms occur, however, epinephrine, not antihistamines, is the necessary treatment for anaphylaxis.

ADDITIONAL MEDICATIONS AND TREATMENTS FOR ANAPHYLAXIS

What additional treatments are given to people having anaphylaxis?
In addition to epinephrine and antihistamines, asthma medications may
be given for those with asthma and wheezing. An emergency room or ambulance has the option to administer various additional treatments, such
as oxygen, intravenous fluids, additional medications to support breathing
and blood pressure, and steroids. The emergency room also has access to
machines that support breathing, if needed.

What type of asthma medications might be given during anaphylaxis?
A bronchodilator, the asthma "rescue" medication that is prescribed to
relieve wheezing from asthma, may be given.

Can a bronchodilator be given for wheezing during anaphylaxis?
It can be given as an *additional* treatment to epinephrine but it CANNOT
be depended on to treat anaphylaxis on its own. Epinephrine is an excellent treatment for wheezing and was a treatment for asthma prior to the
invention of asthma inhalers.

Can a bronchodilator be given in place of epinephrine for anaphylaxis?
Never.

What are steroids?
Corticosteroids are an anti-inflammatory medication that is often given
to reduce wheezing in severe asthma exacerbations. These are different
from the type of steroids abused to build muscle.

When are steroids given for anaphylaxis?
Many physicians will give steroids when there has been a severe allergic
reaction.

Why are steroids given for anaphylaxis?
It is presumed that the steroid will quell later swelling in the lungs, as

they do for asthma exacerbations, and perhaps assist in reducing swelling elsewhere. However, steroids have never been proven to treat symptoms of anaphylaxis.

How long does it take for a steroid to treat symptoms?
Approximately 4 to 6 hours, which underscores why steroids are not part of an immediate emergency plan to treat anaphylaxis as epinephrine is.

Can steroids replace epinephrine to treat anaphylaxis?
Never.

Should I carry steroids to treat anaphylaxis?
Generally, no. They cannot improve symptoms of anaphylaxis and may deter proper therapy. Sometimes physicians prescribe them to carry if a person is going to travel to remote areas, hours away from any medical attention, to presumably assist with the later-onset asthma symptoms of anaphylaxis that sometimes occurs, or to assist in treating a severe asthma exacerbation.

How long should steroids be continued after they are given for anaphylaxis?
Some physicians prescribe them for several days, similar to what is done for an asthma exacerbation, but this approach has not been studied. If there are no further symptoms, a single dose is usually adequate.

What is Singulair (montelukast) and can it be used to treat anaphylaxis?
It is an oral medication used for asthma and hay fever. It blocks one of the inflammatory pathways that is important in allergy, but it has not been studied for treatment of anaphylaxis. It is NOT recommended as a treatment during anaphylaxis.

When waiting for help, how should people undergoing anaphylaxis be treated?
They should be kept calm and be positioned comfortably. This may be a sitting position for a person having trouble breathing. In severe anaphylaxis, particularly if symptoms suggest poor blood circulation, the person

should lie down with legs raised. If he or she is vomiting, however, lying on one side may be safer, to prevent choking.

Why is it suggested to lie down for severe anaphylaxis?

When blood circulation is poor, gravity can pull blood away from important areas of the body, such as the brain and internal organs. Lying with legs raised allows gravity to help get blood where it is needed. Once people with severe anaphylaxis are lying down, they should be kept in this position until they are stabilized by medical experts; there may be danger in standing them up.

Why is it possibly dangerous to sit or stand a person who is having severe anaphylaxis?

If a person has severe anaphylaxis with low blood pressure (anaphylactic shock) and is not fully treated, standing up might pool blood suddenly into the legs, leaving the heart with nothing to pump, which could be fatal. This has rarely been observed to occur in adults.

Does charcoal provide any relief for anaphylaxis?

Activated charcoal (not the kind used in a barbeque) is a medicinal treatment used for poisonings. It has been theorized as a treatment for food anaphylaxis, to absorb the allergen from the gut, but this has not been studied adequately. Although some emergency room physicians may consider this, drawbacks include potential lung damage if the treatment is vomited and accidentally inhaled.

WRITTEN EMERGENCY PLANS, EDUCATION, MEDICAL IDENTIFICATION JEWELRY, MANAGEMENT ISSUES

What is a written emergency plan for anaphylaxis?

These brief written plans, sometimes called anaphylaxis action plans, food allergy emergency plans, and so forth, describe the actions to be taken in the event of an allergic reaction such as anaphylaxis. They are generally created for caregivers of children in schools or camps, but they are helpful for all caregivers and for food-allergic adults as well.

What are the key components of a written food anaphylaxis plan?

The plan identifies the allergic individual (often with a picture), the person's allergies, whether he or she has asthma (a risk for more severe reactions), the typical symptoms to watch for and what treatments to provide if they occur, and contact information. Many plans include additional instructions about the treatments.

Who writes the emergency plan for food allergy?

A physician or a physician's qualified assistant.

Where can I find a written food allergy emergency action plan?

If your doctor or school does not have their own, you can download one from a variety of websites (see the resources in chapter 11).

What is medical identification jewelry?

This is a bracelet or pendant that has a medical insignia and describes the medical condition and potential severe risks, for example, food allergy and anaphylaxis.

Why is medical identification jewelry recommended?

In the event the victim becomes incapacitated during a reaction, this can inform passers-by and medical professionals. For children, this may also be a helpful reminder to others about not offering unsafe foods.

Where do I get medical identification jewelry?

Several companies make them. The largest one is a not-for-profit foundation, MedicAlert (www.medicalert.org). You may want to list some of your food allergies and indicate "anaphylaxis" or just indicate "food allergy and anaphylaxis." This foundation also has an option to keep your personal medical information on file so that a responder can get additional details by contacting MedicAlert.

What are additional ways to have notification about allergies?
The cell phone has become a fixture for most people. Having allergy notification there can be an additional help. You can use ICE.

How do you get a cell phone to show emergency information and what is ICE?
ICE stands for "In Case of Emergency." Various cell phone apps allow
your cell phone or smartphone to call emergency services, present medical information, and alert responders about medical problems, including
food allergies. Cell phone service providers may also offer an ICE icon.
At minimum, an ICE contact can be created using ICE ahead of the name
(for example, ICE-mothercellnumber), and the specific medical problems
such as allergies can be added in the notes field.

What other aspects of medical care should a person at risk for food anaphy-
laxis address?
Keeping asthma under good control.

Why is it important to keep asthma in good control for people at risk of food
anaphylaxis?
It is presumed that a vulnerable lung increases the risk of having breathing problems during anaphylaxis. Although having stable, well-controlled
asthma is still a risk factor, it is more dangerous to have anaphylaxis when
the lung is already wheezing and swelling.

Delving Deeper:
PREDICTING ANAPHYLAXIS AND TAKING A TREATMENT QUIZ

What is on the horizon for better prediction of food anaphylaxis?
Unfortunately, current allergy tests are not good at predicting severity.
This is not a surprise since the test does not know your other risk factors,
for example, how much food might be eaten or if you also have asthma.
Studies are under way to develop tests that are able to predict severity bet-
ter, for example, by determining which food proteins or segments of pro-

teins the immune system is attacking. Another strategy being investigated is to evaluate a person's baseline metabolism for specific chemicals and allergic mediators, because these may alter the strength of the person's allergic response. One example under study is an enzyme that destroys a chemical called platelet-activating factor (PAF), which is released during an allergic reaction.

How do I know if I should inject epinephrine?

If you are ever in doubt, it is better to inject. The medication is safe and was used routinely as an asthma treatment before inhaled asthma medications were in widespread use. To get a better idea of when to respond with epinephrine, try this quiz, where I ask *you* the questions.

Consider the following scenarios and decide whether epinephrine or some other medication (such as antihistamines or asthma inhalers) are the best choice. Compare your answers to mine at the end of this chapter.

Situation 1. A child with a peanut allergy ate a peanut a minute ago and now has three hives on her face and no other symptoms:

   a) Inject epinephrine and give antihistamine

   b) Give antihistamine and watch

Situation 2. Your 16-year-old child care assistant calls you to say that your 3-year-old child, who is severely allergic to milk, eggs, and peanuts and has had severe reactions in the past, may have eaten something he is allergic to because he has hives on his face. The sitter does not think he is coughing or having any other problems, but he stopped playing with his ball. What should you tell her to do?

   a) Inject epinephrine and give antihistamine

   b) Give antihistamine and watch

Situation 3. You are in a bakery with your 18-month-old in your arms. She is allergic to peanuts. While you are eyeing a cake, she grabs a cookie, which you know because you hear chewing and see crumbs spilling from her full mouth. You jostle her and in a panic scream, "How did you grab that?" She immediately stops breathing and is turning blue.

a) Inject epinephrine and give antihistamine

b) Give antihistamine and watch

c) Do something else

Situation 4. Your child, who has milk and egg allergies, ate a safe lunch. He also has asthma and has been developing a cold. He went to play outside and came back inside with a hacking cough and wheezing. He has no other symptoms.

a) Inject epinephrine and give antihistamine

b) Give antihistamine and watch

c) Give an asthma inhaler (bronchodilator)

Situation 5. A child with severe egg allergy is finger painting. She develops an itchy eye that swells shut while she is rubbing it. There are no other symptoms. The teacher realizes that she had smoothed the paint with egg white.

a) Inject epinephrine and give antihistamine

b) Give antihistamine and watch

Situation 6. A 19-year-old girl has a severe peanut allergy. She is carrying her self-injectable epinephrine. Her friend opens a bag of potato chips, and after eating a few, she asks if it is okay that they are flavored with peanut oil and that she is eating them in the same room. The girl with peanut allergy says that she feels like she is having trouble breathing. She looks pale. She says her fingers feel numb and she might vomit. What should she do?

a) Inject epinephrine and take antihistamine

b) Take antihistamine and watch

c) Do something else

Also of Interest:
EXERCISE AND ANAPHYLAXIS

What are the theories about why food-associated exercise-induced anaphylaxis (FAEIA) happens?

FAEIA is a condition where a food that is otherwise tolerated causes anaphylaxis if a person exercises after eating it. One theory to explain this is that exercise may alter gut blood flow, allowing certain proteins to be absorbed more readily into the bloodstream. Another theory is that exercise activates gut enzymes that may alter proteins in a way that makes them more visible to the immune system, resulting in reactions.

ANSWERS TO DELVING DEEPER: ANAPHYLAXIS TREATMENT QUIZ

1. ANSWER: Either choice could be correct. It would likely depend on knowing more about the child. If the child has had extremely severe past reactions to peanuts, with breathing problems, for example, one might go ahead and use the epinephrine. If past reactions were all mild skin rashes, it would be reasonable to give antihistamines and watch carefully.

2. ANSWER: I would suggest giving the epinephrine. In this case, it is a concern that an inexperienced person is making the decisions. The child already has hives, is behaving differently, and the 16-year-old may not be able to monitor the reaction appropriately. The child is also known to have multiple severe allergies and apparently ate something that was an allergen. I think the best decision is to have the sitter inject epinephrine and call 911.

3. ANSWER: You may have chosen to inject epinephrine because there is a breathing problem. However, this is a bit of a trick question. An allergic reaction should not result in an inability to breathe seconds after eating the allergen. That would just be too fast for an allergic reaction. Here, the baby had a mouth full of cookie and was jostled. Most likely, she is choking and needs a Heimlich maneuver to dislodge the cookie from her windpipe.

4. ANSWER: Although wheezing and coughing suggest the need to treat a food-allergic reaction with epinephrine, this child has asthma and has two reasons to wheeze: his respiratory infection and exercise. He also ate a safe lunch, so there is no suggestion that he ate a food to which he is allergic. Therefore, giving an asthma inhaler is the best choice. If you did give this child epinephrine, it would also help his wheezing.

5. ANSWER: It is most reasonable to give antihistamines and watch. There is no evidence that the girl ate the egg-laden paint, but she did rub it in her eye. The eye is sensitive and swells easily. For example, people with pollen allergy may experience significant eyelid swelling just from pollen in the air. It is not likely that a skin or an eye exposure will progress to anaphylaxis.

6. ANSWER: The girl is describing problems affecting her gut, breathing, and possibly circulation. These would normally suggest anaphylaxis, and it is prudent to respond by giving epinephrine, but it is probably unnecessary in this case. Her symptoms also match those of anxiety and hyperventilation (breathing fast, hard, and heavy). It is most likely that the girl is nervous about being near the peanut oil and is having a panic attack. This response is common because people react with anxiety to something they know can hurt them. Imagine having a gun to the head. You might breathe heavy and faint, but that is not an allergy.

Hyperventilating causes imbalances in blood acids that result in feeling light-headed and in finger tingling or numbness. She might benefit from being calmed and breathing into a bag; however, given the uncertainty in the moment, it may be reasonable to inject epinephrine and sort out the circumstances later. In this case, not injecting epinephrine is reasonable because there are many reasons to suspect there is no allergic reaction: anaphylaxis is not likely from air exposure, peanut oil often has no proteins from peanut, and even if the oil had peanut protein, it would not permeate the air. The final decision would probably depend on the confidence of an observer, but if the girl was the person deciding to inject, I would suggest that she go ahead and do so.

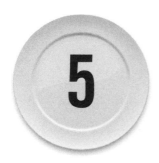

What **CHRONIC HEALTH PROBLEMS** Are Caused by Food Allergy?

This chapter includes answers to questions about several chronic illnesses that are caused by food allergy. I describe how chronic allergic symptoms may be related to foods and discuss medical conditions that are not so clearly related to food allergies.

GENERAL QUESTIONS ABOUT CHRONIC ILLNESSES AND FOODS

Can food allergies cause symptoms that are persistent (chronic) rather than sudden after a food is eaten?
Yes. Many chronic skin and gastrointestinal illnesses are associated with food allergies.

What chronic allergic illnesses can be related to food allergies?
Food allergy can contribute to atopic dermatitis and various gastrointestinal illnesses in infants, children, and adults.

RESPIRATORY SYMPTOMS

Is asthma caused by food allergies?
Generally not. Triggers of asthma include respiratory infections, exercise, and allergens in the air, such as pollens, dust mites, and animal danders. During a severe allergic reaction to food, asthma may flare. Studies suggest that it is uncommon for ingestion of a food to lead to the chronic lung inflammation that causes asthma. For some people with chronic asthma, however, food allergy does play a role.

How often does food allergy contribute to chronic asthma?
Various studies of people with asthma show that foods contribute to asthma episodes in fewer than 1 in 25 asthmatic children and even less frequently among adults. Even so, isolated chronic asthma, without food allergy, skin reactions, or gut symptoms, is rare.

How can I tell if my asthma is caused by food allergies?
The first assumption should be that they are not related. If there is a strong suspicion, however, and the asthma is not responding well to medical treatments, testing can be done. If testing is positive, it would likely require a trial period of avoiding the suspected food and then reintroducing it, under medical supervision, to see if there is a relationship.

Is hay fever caused by food allergies?
Generally not. Nasal symptoms itching, sneezing, runny nose, and congestion—are common during a food-allergic reaction, but chronic hay fever is typically attributable to allergens in the air, such as pollens.

HIVES

Are chronic hives, those occurring almost daily for many weeks, caused by food allergies?

Usually not. A few studies suggest that the chemical nature of food additives may contribute to chronic hives in fewer than 5% of cases. As a chemical effect, this is not an allergy. True food allergies are rarely related to chronic hives.

Why would food allergy not be a likely cause of chronic hives?

Hives are the most common symptoms of an allergic reaction to food, but they typically occur in minutes and fade within an hour of eating the causal food. They do not recur unless the food is eaten again. People with an illness called "chronic urticaria," or chronic hives, have the rash on most days for over six weeks. It would be quite odd for a person to eat the causal food, experience hives, and then eat the food again and again without realizing a connection.

What is the cause of chronic urticaria?

When someone has hives for a week or two, the most common trigger is a viral infection. If the hives are unrelenting for many weeks, they are most often due to a type of autoimmune response, when the body is attacking its own allergy cells. This is different from hives that are caused by food allergy, that occur soon after the food is eaten, resolve quickly, and do not recur unless the food is eaten again. People with chronic hives have a higher rate of making antibodies against molecules on their allergy cells, hence activating them to cause hives. These individuals are also at risk to develop other illnesses where the body is attacking itself, for example, thyroid problems.

Is food ever a contributing factor to chronic hives?

There are theories that some components of foods might cause or contribute to chronic hives. A few studies suggest that chemicals in foods might cause hives in some people. Because the theory is not about an allergic reaction, the term "pseudoallergen" has been used.

What are pseudoallergens?

According to this theory, food additives, vasoactive substances such as histamine, and some natural substances in fruits, vegetables, and spices contribute to chronic hives. A trial of a pseudoallergen-free diet is recommended by proponents of this theory.

What is involved with a pseudoallergen-free diet?

The list of foods to avoid is extensive. One group suggests avoiding the following: chewing gum, candy, and similar products; spices and herbs (except salt and chives); additives—E100–E1518, preservatives and artificial colors, gelling agents, thickening matter, humectant, emulsifiers, flavor potentiators, antioxidants, separating agents, sweeteners, baking agents, modified starches, foaming agents, stabilizers, flavoring agents; breads with additional grains, herbs, or other such added ingredients; alcohol; sesame; eggs and pasta with eggs; cake; biscuits; potato chips; margarine and mayonnaise; smoked meats; seafood; tomatoes, artichokes, peas, mushrooms, spinach, rhubarb, olives, sweet peppers; dried fruits and fruit juices; and herbal tea. The diet allows only fresh foods—no preserved foods, except deep-frozen foods without any additives.

How long is the pseudoallergen-free diet for chronic hives to be tried?

Three weeks.

What is the success rate of the pseudoallergen-free diet for chronic hives?

One group claims a success rate of one in six, with up to one in three having some improvement.

Is a pseudoallergen-free diet for chronic hives recommended?

There are only a few studies and no large studies comparing people who tried the diet to those who did not. Some researchers claim that the diet might cure the hives because after many months, the foods could be added back without recurrence of hives. I am suspicious that without a comparison group treated with a placebo diet, the effect of this extensive diet is unproven. Some of the people treated would likely have resolved their hives after weeks or months whether or not they followed the diet. The diet is healthful, though, so I would not deter a person from trying it. It should be done in coordination with a physician, however, and after discussing the nature of the illness, standard treatments, and consideration of alternative causes of chronic hives (and associated illnesses as discussed above).

ATOPIC DERMATITIS (ECZEMA)

What is atopic dermatitis?

Atopic dermatitis, more generally called eczema, is a skin condition. The main symptom is an itchy rash that tends to run in families; occurs in people with other allergic problems, such as asthma; and follows a pattern on the skin that varies by age. For infants, the scalp, face, chest, arms, and legs are often affected. Children and adults tend to have the rashes in the folds of the knees, elbows, and neck, along with other areas.

What causes atopic dermatitis?

Many different triggers inflame the hyper-irritable skin of someone with eczema. The skin is also prone to infection and has a defective barrier, so it dries out easily.

Is eczema caused by food allergies?

There is some controversy about whether foods can contribute to the chronic rashes of atopic dermatitis. About one in three children with more than mild atopic dermatitis have food allergies, including anaphylaxis. Because there are many other triggers, how many children's eczema is primarily due to food allergy is unclear. Some children (and much less frequently adults) do clearly have food-related flaring of their atopic dermatitis.

What triggers eczema/atopic dermatitis other than food?

The primary triggers are irritants, such as sweating, dryness, soaps, scratching, clothing that holds in moisture or is itchy like wool; infections; stress; and allergens from the environment, such as animal danders and pollens.

How is atopic dermatitis treated?

Treatment may require hydrating baths (long soaks in lukewarm water); application of topical medications that reduce inflammation, such as steroids and other anti-inflammatory creams or ointments; antibiotics to reduce infection; and moisturizers and creams to improve the skin barrier. Irritants are reduced by using mild soaps or by double rinsing clothes and using cotton rather than wool or polyester. Nails kept short will reduce scratching. Antihistamines may be used to lessen itching and to induce sedation at bedtime, which further minimizes scratching.

How is food allergy related to eczema / atopic dermatitis?

Some studies show that removal of a particular food allergen can help relieve symptoms and that the symptoms increase when the food is returned to the diet (unless the allergies are outgrown).

Which foods may contribute to eczema / atopic dermatitis?

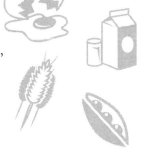

The most likely triggers for children are eggs, milk, wheat, and soy.

What are the benefits of identifying and removing foods to treat eczema / atopic dermatitis?

There may be improved control of the rash.

What are the risks of removing foods that may contribute to eczema / atopic dermatitis?

There are several. Avoiding foods carries nutritional risks and affects social interactions. Removing a food that is a stable part of the diet but that tests positively as an allergy can rarely result in the allergy being more immediate and severe when the food is encountered. Although this is an uncommon occurrence, it is the reason medical treatments should be tried and maximized prior to removing foods. This is discussed further in chapter 3.

Who with atopic dermatitis should be tested for food allergies?

Experts have suggested that food allergies should be considered for people with atopic dermatitis who have noticed allergic reactions to foods or flaring of their eczema rash with foods. Another group that may warrant an investigation for food allergy are children under age 5 who have more than mild atopic dermatitis and whose rash is not responding well to standard treatments. A good skin care treatment regimen should be tried before considering food allergies, however, because removal of foods from the diet carries nutritional, social, and possibly immunological consequences (as explained above).

How does one identify what foods may contribute to atopic dermatitis?

Assuming the eczema rash did not respond well to medical treatments, foods can be considered as possible triggers. Typically, tests are performed to identify possible triggers, focusing on the few foods that are most often the cause. The suspected food is removed for a few weeks and returned to the diet under medical supervision. See chapter 3 for more details about diagnosis.

How easy is it to determine which foods might be contributing to atopic dermatitis?

It is extremely difficult. In studies of children with atopic dermatitis, most of the foods the family and patient suspected to be triggering the rash were disproven as triggers.

Why is it difficult to determine which foods contribute to atopic dermatitis?

There are two reasons. First, atopic dermatitis has a naturally waxing and waning course, which can be misleading when trying to make causal connections to foods. To make matters worse, some studies suggest that the symptoms can arise in the day or two after the food is eaten. This means that if you add a food, any flaring of the eczema in the next day or two could be attributed to the food when in reality the rash might have naturally flared.

The second hurdle is that atopic dermatitis improves from medical management but is not cured. This means that a few days of skin care may significantly improve the rash, only to have it flare up when treatments are withdrawn. Often there is reluctance to treat with medications, and treatments are stopped when the rash improves. This approach is often doomed because the medication is stopped and the trialed food is started at the same time. This can lead to the false impression that the food caused the flare when really the lack of continued medical treatment was the reason. Trials of adding foods to the diet should be undertaken during consistent treatment and when the skin is in good repair.

What is the suggested approach to determine if foods are contributing to eczema?

The fundamental diagnostic tests described in chapter 3 (medical history, skin tests, blood tests, oral food challenges) should be administered. It is important not to change the daily treatment regimen while trials of food elimination and oral food challenge are undertaken. If the skin responds extremely well to medical therapy, it is beneficial to work with your doctor to attain the best management with the least amount of medication, perhaps in lieu of removing foods if this is achievable. Recall that atopic dermatitis is a skin disorder and that there are many triggers. However, if management with skin treatments is failing and a food is the cause, removal from the diet can be helpful.

GASTROINTESTINAL, DIGESTIVE ILLNESSES

What stomach, digestive, or intestinal symptoms are triggered by foods?

The gut experiences only a few symptoms: pain, heartburn (acid reflux), nausea, vomiting, diarrhea, and poor nutrient absorption, leading to weight loss, poor weight gain, or growth failure. Foods can cause these symptoms due to an allergy or other reasons. Most gut problems, however, are not due to a food allergy.

Can chronic gut symptoms be attributed to foods?

Unlike most symptoms of a food allergy, where symptoms happen soon after a food is eaten and resolve fairly quickly afterward, chronic gut symptoms are not so clearly related to particular meals. For example, a person may be experiencing frequent pain, vomiting, and diarrhea that does not simply follow specific meals.

What kinds of symptoms are likely when foods are causing chronic allergic gut symptoms?
The most common symptoms include stomach pain, pain with swallowing, nausea, vomiting, diarrhea (especially with blood), heartburn / reflux, and poor weight gain or growth.

When should gut symptoms alert a person that there is a food allergy?
There are two ways: (1) when symptoms of pain, nausea, vomiting, or diarrhea occur soon after a meal; and (2) when symptoms have characteristics often seen in food allergies that affect the gut. These symptoms are consistent with a diagnosis of medical disorders called proctocolitis, enterocolitis, and eosinophilic gut disease.

COLIC, CONSTIPATION, IRRITABLE BOWEL SYNDROME, AND REFLUX

What is infant colic?
Colic is defined by frequent long periods of inconsolable crying. The strict medical definition of colic requires that an otherwise healthy infant show unexplained fussing or crying for over three hours a day, more than three days a week, for longer than three weeks. Most parents, however, would consider their infant to be "colicky" with much less intense or extended periods of crying. Remember too that there may be medical reasons for inconsolable crying, anything from severe gut disease to having a hair stuck around a finger or toe, so always discuss this with your doctor.

Is infant colic due to food allergy?
Although some studies have linked foods as a contributing factor, food al-

lergy is not a typical trigger. The rate of colic seems to be similar whether infants are breast fed or formula fed, although some studies suggest colic is less frequent among those breast fed. A baby with severe atopic dermatitis (eczema) and gastrointestinal symptoms like diarrhea may indeed have a food allergy and may be irritable and crying in relation to these symptoms. This is not an "otherwise healthy" infant, so this type of discomfort should not be considered true colic.

What treatments should be considered for colic?
Overall, no convincing studies prove any approach to be effective in reducing colic. Anti-gas medications do not appear to work. Reducing stimulation of the infant, according to several studies, helps 50% of infants with colic or reduces symptoms by about 50%. Some studies support dietary approaches. Any approaches to colic should be done in communication with your pediatrician or allergist.

Should the mother's diet be altered if there is colic?
Some studies show that when a breast-feeding mother avoids or reduces her consumption of milk, colic may improve whether or not there are other signs of milk allergy. Various studies have evaluated low-allergen diets, when a mother avoids typical allergenic foods (such as milk and eggs) while breast feeding. In general, this approach was sometimes effective, but it remains unproved. Dietary changes are generally not advised as a first step in addressing colic.

Should the infant's diet be altered if there is colic?
Switching a colicky infant to a hypoallergenic infant formula may result in improved colic, whether or not there are signs of milk allergy, according to some studies. Others suggest that a lactose-free formula may be helpful. Some evidence supports using a soy formula or even an herbal tea (though use of a tea in infants can cause nutritional deficits). In general, the low-allergen diet was effective, but only about one-half to one-third as effective as reducing stimulation (see above). Dietary changes are generally unproved as treatments for colic and are not a first step.

What dietary approaches are suggested for colic if reduced stimulation doesn't work?

Although studies are lacking, some suggest treatment with reduced stimulation and then, if needed, a weeklong trial on a low-allergen diet. In any event, a link to allergy has not been proved. Colic improves spontaneously, so luckily there is an end in sight even if these dietary measures do not seem to work.

What is constipation?

Constipation is a symptom that describes having infrequent bowel movements, possibly hard stools, and possibly painful defecation. There are a huge number of potential causes, including diet, medications, diseases of the bowel, and psychological issues.

Is constipation due to food allergy?

A few studies link milk allergy to constipation that has not responded to other measures. By far, however, most constipation is not related to food allergies.

How is diet related to constipation?

Talk to your doctor if you are experiencing constipation. Dietary measures, such as increasing fiber or liquids, may be recommended.

What is irritable bowel syndrome?

Abbreviated IBS, this syndrome is diagnosed when there is a failure to identify medical illnesses contributing to a constellation of symptoms that include stomach pain, discomfort, and either constipation or diarrhea. Different subtypes are identified. Some include mostly diarrhea, others constipation, and others alternating constipation and diarrhea. Sometimes the illness develops after an infection. IBS tends to be chronic and affects quality of life.

What causes irritable bowel syndrome?

There are many theories about the causes, from infections to stress. Your doctor should consider medical illnesses that could cause the symptoms, including infection, celiac disease, and inflammatory bowel diseases. Treatments include medications, psychotherapy, probiotics, and dietary alterations.

Is irritable bowel syndrome caused by food allergies?
Food allergy is one problem to consider when an individual experiences some of the symptoms of IBS. No studies specifically identify food allergy as a cause of the syndrome itself. Nonetheless, if symptoms such as pain and vomiting occur consistently and soon after eating specific foods, the evaluations described in chapter 3 may be warranted. For IBS, however, the terms food "sensitivity" or "intolerance" are sometimes used because dietary alterations can improve IBS symptoms despite absence of true allergy.

What role does food play in irritable bowel syndrome?
A number of studies have tried to use various elimination diets, some with success, although careful studies are lacking. Gluten-free diets in particular have helped some persons with IBS. Contributing problems of lactose intolerance or other sugar intolerances may be responsible. Eliminating some foods, such as milk or wheat, may result in increasing other foods that promote better digestion, such as fruits and vegetables. It appears that supplementation with soluble fiber, such as psyllium, can improve the symptoms for many sufferers. Insoluble fiber such as cellulose may be unhelpful. Discuss any diet or medication with your health care professional.

Can IgG tests identify foods causing IBS?
As discussed in chapter 3, IgG or IgG4 is a normal immune response to foods. Studies have not convincingly shown that such testing can identify food triggers in IBS. Although dietary alterations may be one means to address IBS (along with fiber, medications, stress reduction, and so on), these specific tests are not proved.

What is reflux?
Also known as gastroesophageal reflux disease (GERD), or acid reflux, this illness occurs when stomach acid comes up into the esophagus, the tube

connecting the mouth and stomach. Symptoms can include heartburn, cough, chest pain, and pain with or trouble swallowing. The acid can burn the esophagus and may come up into the throat and nose causing asthma, hoarseness, tooth decay, sinus troubles, and chronic damage to the esophagus.

What causes reflux?

Reflux is usually attributed to problems that make it easier for food and acid to make it up past the valve that usually prevents a backwash from the stomach. For example, there may be a physical problem with this valve, or obesity may lead to increased pressure, or medications or illnesses may reduce the strength of the valve. There may be overproduction of stomach acid as well.

Is reflux due to food allergy?

Reflux is usually not caused by food allergies, although a few studies have shown a link for some people, especially to milk in children. Another illness that is a concern with reflux symptoms is eosinophilic esophagitis, an allergic disorder often associated with food allergies. This illness sometimes mimics reflux, but certain symptoms differentiate it, as described later in this chapter.

CELIAC DISEASE (GLUTEN-SENSITIVE ENTEROPATHY)

What is celiac disease?

Celiac disease is caused by an immune system response to gluten, a protein in wheat, and related proteins in barley and rye. The disorder is also called gluten-sensitive enteropathy. This is an inherited disorder affecting the gut and sometimes other parts of the body. Nearly 1 in 100 persons has celiac disease.

Is celiac disease a food allergy?

Although celiac disease is caused by an abnormal immune response to gluten, most people do not consider this to be a typical food allergy because the symptoms are so different.

How does celiac disease differ from a wheat allergy?

Wheat allergy results in rapid, typical symptoms of allergy, such as hives and swelling. Unfortunately, unlike most food allergies, celiac disease symptoms are chronic, and the disease does not resolve. Celiac disease is also associated with a risk for cancer.

When is celiac disease suspected?

The diagnosis of celiac disease is considered if there are symptoms such as diarrhea, poor growth, stomach pain, vomiting, constipation, bloating, and irritability. Since this disease is inherited, suspicion is higher if other family members have celiac disease. Sometimes there are symptoms outside of the gut, for example, poorly developed tooth enamel, blistering skin rashes, and poor bone development.

How is celiac disease diagnosed?

Blood tests can be done if a person is currently eating gluten-containing grains. Genetic testing may also help determine a diagnosis. The most accurate method of diagnosis requires a biopsy of the gut.

How is celiac disease treated?

By strict avoidance of gluten.

PROCTOCOLITIS (FOOD PROTEIN–INDUCED PROCTOCOLITIS)

My infant has mucousy, bloody stools. Is this a food allergy?

It may be a food allergy called food protein–induced proctocolitis.

What is proctocolitis?

Proctocolitis, or food protein–induced proctocolitis, is the name of a food allergy affecting infants that causes the stool to have mucous and blood. It is most often diagnosed in breast-fed babies. These babies are otherwise well, are growing normally, do not have other symptoms, and do not become anemic because the amount of blood lost is usually small.

Is food allergy the only reason a baby might have bloody or mucousy stools?

No. This symptom can also result from infections; anatomical problems, such as blockages; or minor irritations, such as small tears in the anus. Babies with proctocolitis have stool with small amounts of mucous and blood mixed in, whereas some of the other problems may result in diarrhea (infection) or a small bit of blood on the surface of a stool (tear). If you see blood in the stool, talk to your doctor; do not assume it is proctocolitis.

What causes proctocolitis?

Proctocolitis is a minor allergic response to a protein, such as cow's milk protein in infant formulas or passed in the mother's breast milk. The illness is generally mild, and the baby is otherwise well. If a biopsy is performed, a small amount of allergic inflammation is seen in the rectum, but a biopsy is rarely needed.

What foods trigger proctocolitis?

By far the most common trigger is cow's milk. Other potential causes include soy, eggs, wheat, and others.

How is proctocolitis treated?

For breast-fed infants, the mother is usually instructed to avoid or reduce cow's milk in her diet. The bleeding should stop within a few days. If it continues, other foods may be avoided, and the doctor may look harder for other causes.

Does the mother of an infant with proctocolitis have to strictly avoid the food?

Not necessarily. When first removing a food from the diet, it should be removed strictly to see if the bleeding responds. After that, the mother may be able to have small amounts in her diet without producing symptoms in the infant.

Does food-allergic proctocolitis go away?
Yes.

How long does it take for food-allergic proctocolitis to resolve?
Depending on how severe the symptoms were, tests for resolution might be made in weeks or a few months after the symptoms respond to dietary elimination. The course of resolution has not been studied adequately, but proctocolitis is usually resolved by the time an infant is 1 year old. Some studies suggest that a virus is often the true cause of bleeding, which argues for adding the suspected trigger food back sooner to see if the bleeding is truly related to the food.

How do you know if food-allergic proctocolitis has resolved?
Your physician will simply instruct you to gradually add milk (or other trigger foods) to your diet if you are still breast feeding or to the infant's diet. If you see blood reappear, then avoidance is resumed until the next trial.

Do infants with proctocolitis go on to have other food allergies?
They are not at significantly higher risk.

FOOD PROTEIN–INDUCED ENTEROCOLITIS SYNDROME

My infant had severe vomiting two hours after a meal, became pale and sleepy, and later had diarrhea. Is that a food allergy?
It may be a food allergy called food protein–induced enterocolitis syndrome (FPIES).

What is FPIES?
This is a serious food allergy that usually starts in infancy. The symptoms are severe vomiting and diarrhea. Unlike typical food allergies, there are no hives or wheezing, and allergy tests by skin or blood are negative.

How would I know if my infant has FPIES?

There is a typical pattern of symptoms that differ depending on whether the food has been a consistent part of the diet or was ingested after a period of avoidance. FPIES is often initially misdiagnosed as an infection, with consideration of a food allergy coming up when repeated symptoms are noted from reintroduction of the trigger foods.

What are the symptoms of FPIES when a baby is routinely eating the food that causes the reaction?

The infant will have increasing vomiting and diarrhea and may appear pale and lethargic. He or she can seem very ill, and physicians might suspect a serious infection or surgical problem.

What are the symptoms of FPIES from first ingestion of a food or from reintroducing it after not eating it for a time?

The infant or young child appears perfectly well for about one to three hours but then begins to vomit, often profusely and repetitively. The child may become pale or blue in color and lethargic, with low blood pressure. Several hours later there is often diarrhea. The illness looks very much like a severe infection. If a blood test is performed, there may be a large number of cells called neutrophils and a high number of platelets, another blood component. The blood test results may lead a doctor to further suspect infection.

What foods cause FPIES?

The most common foods are milk and soy. When grains are responsible, usually oat or rice is the allergen. Many different foods have been found to trigger this response in children.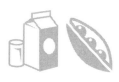

What are the chances that a baby with milk FPIES will react to other foods?

This varies a lot among study findings, but roughly half of these children react to soy, and about a quarter of them react to a solid food, such as oat or rice.

What are the chances that a baby with rice or oat FPIES will react to other solids?

More than half the patients in our referral center react to more than one food, with about two-thirds reacting to milk or soy and about half reacting to another grain (not usually wheat). These percentages have been much lower in studies from other countries. It means that advancing the diet requires care and working with an allergist.

How is FPIES treated?

The only current treatment is to avoid the trigger foods.

Why does FPIES happen?

The immune system responds to trigger foods by releasing chemicals affecting the gut and circulation. These are somewhat different from those that are released in anaphylaxis. IgE is not involved.

How is an FPIES reaction treated?

The primary treatment is to avoid the trigger food. If the food is eaten and a reaction occurs, the child should be given fluids. Because blood pressure is often low, and the child is vomiting, fluids are given through a vein (intravenously, an IV) under medical supervision. Therefore, treatment in an emergency room is required. The reaction is thought to be due to immune cells, so treatment with steroids to quell immune cells is also usually given, but this treatment is not proved. Medicines used for anaphylaxis, such as epinephrine and antihistamines, are not typically used.

Should a child with FPIES have epinephrine available?

I usually prescribe self-injectable epinephrine to have on hand for FPIES. The usefulness of this medication may be limited, however, because the main concern is to restore fluids. Parents would not use this treatment unless the child was very ill and delayed in getting to a health care provider for fluids.

Are there different severities of FPIES?
Yes, an FPIES reaction may be mild, with just a small amount of vomiting, or severe, with all the symptoms described above.

Can FPIES be fatal?
Thus far, there have been no recorded deaths attributed to FPIES.

How do you approach feeding new foods to a baby who has FPIES?
Because there is currently no simple test to predict a reaction, introduction of the most common triggers (milk, soy, oat, rice) is often delayed until the infant is age 1 year or older. We do not know if there is any benefit to waiting longer, or possibly trying sooner, however, so this should be individualized with your allergist.

How are decisions about introducing new foods made for infants with FPIES?
This can be complicated. Your allergist has to decide whether foods can be tried at home or should be introduced under supervision, and when. The timing of introducing risky foods might vary depending on the severity of past reactions—waiting longer, for example, if past reactions were severe. The decisions are also based on epidemiology, or the risk for particular foods. Introducing oat or rice for the first time to an infant who already reacted to milk and soy is riskier than trying other foods (fruits, vegetables, meats, and other grains). If an infant had reactions to foods that are rare triggers (sweet potatoes, other vegetables, fruits), going slower and more cautiously with more introductions under supervision would be warranted.

Does FPIES resolve?
In most cases it does.

How is an infant or child tested to see if FPIES has resolved?
By a feeding test. Allergy patch tests have been tried as a form of diagnosis but with mixed results. See chapter 3 for more details about these methods.

How long does it take for FPIES to go away?

It is difficult to test for resolution because a feeding test is needed. The problem appears to resolve in one to three years in most cases.

Can a baby with FPIES develop "regular" food allergies?

Yes, about 10% of the time. Even though typical tests for allergies do not give any information about whether FPIES has resolved, they might be performed to check if typical anaphylactic allergies have developed.

What should I do if my child is having symptoms or has eaten a food that triggered FPIES in the past?

You should go to the emergency room even before the symptoms start, if possible. Since many doctors are not completely familiar with FPIES, I suggest carrying a letter that explains the illness. Here is an example letter:

Dear Doctor [or To Whom It May Concern],

My child has a food allergy called food protein–induced enterocolitis syndrome. This is a type of allergy that usually does not result in typical allergic symptoms such as hives or wheezing; instead it has isolated gastrointestinal symptoms.

    The foods that my child is avoiding include: _____ .

The symptoms of this type of allergic reaction include repetitive vomiting, which may not start until a few hours (e.g., 2) following ingestion of the food to which my child is allergic. Even trace amounts can trigger a reaction. There is often diarrhea that starts later (after 6 hours). In some cases (~20%), the reaction includes hypotension and lethargy, sometimes acidemia and methemoglobinemia. The treatment is symptomatic and can include intravenous fluids (e.g., normal saline bolus, hydration) and steroids for significant symptoms. The latter is given because the pathophysiology is that of a T-cell response.

    This information is being given for consideration in the differential diagnosis of my child in the event of symptoms. Of course, my child having this illness does not preclude the possibility of other illnesses (e.g., infection, toxic ingestion, etc.) or even other types of allergic reactions leading to symptoms, so it is up to the evaluating physician to consider all possibilities. Similarly, the treating physician is encouraged to pursue any other treatments deemed necessary (e.g., symptomatic, such as epinephrine for shock, antibiotics for presumed infection, etc.).

Sincerely,
Your name [or your doctor's name]

The letter has a lot of "doctor speak," which I will decode: *acidemia* is increased acid in the blood, *hypotension* is low blood pressure, *T-cells* are mentioned to explain that this is not an IgE antibody–related allergy, and *methemoglobinemia* is a response leading to blue color of the skin.

Can a breast-fed baby have FPIES from food eaten by the mother?

This happens rarely. If it does, the mother must avoid eating the causal food.

Does a mother who is breast feeding need to avoid the food that triggered FPIES in her infant when the baby ate the food directly?

We do not have studies comparing outcomes whether a mother avoids the food or not. Assuming the infant is otherwise doing well, I do not usually have a mother avoid the culprit food, but I may advise her not to exceed the amounts she has usually eaten while the infant has been well.

How much food must be eaten by an infant or child to trigger an FPIES reaction?

Similar to typical allergies, some children may be sensitive to trace amounts, and others might not react until ingesting a larger amount. There is no test to see how sensitive a child might be. Sometimes we see a child tolerate an increasing amount prior to having symptoms as they outgrow the allergy.

Can an FPIES reaction be triggered from touch or smell?

No.

Can FPIES occur in adults?

Yes, but it is uncommon. It may occur because an allergy was never outgrown (rare) or occur in response to a food that is a common allergen in adults, such as seafood.

Does FPIES run in families?

There are insufficient studies to know for certain, but siblings may have a higher risk.

FOOD PROTEIN ENTEROPATHY AND PROTEIN INTOLERANCE

What is food protein enteropathy?

This is an uncommon illness of infants with some symptoms similar to celiac disease (diarrhea, poor growth, and low protein, or loss of protein in the gut). There can be swelling of the face and body because of protein imbalances. If a gastroenterologist does a biopsy, inflammation is seen in the gut. Unlike celiac, this illness resolves. The common triggers are milk or soy.

What is food protein intolerance?

The term "food protein intolerance" is not defined in any specific way; it is not a medical diagnosis. It is sometimes used to describe FPIES, eosinophilic gastroenteropathy, or nonspecific gastrointestinal symptoms that are attributed to foods.

EOSINOPHILIC ESOPHAGITIS AND OTHER EOSINOPHILIC GUT DISEASES

What is an eosinophil?

An eosinophil is a cell of the immune system that is prominent in the allergic inflammation that causes asthma and chronic allergic inflammation in the gut.

Food gets stuck in the throat or hurts going down after being swallowed. Can this be a food allergy?

This symptom is a common one in older children and adults who have eosinophilic esophagitis, an illness often related to food allergies.

What is eosinophilic esophagitis?

This is a chronic illness in which allergic inflammation, comprising eosinophils, occurs in the esophagus, the tube that squeezes food from the mouth into the stomach. The esophagus is the most common location of this type of inflammation in the gut. The illness is tough to treat because it is like having a rash inside the body. It is hard to know what is triggering inflammation or how it responds to treatments. Some people may develop scarring that seriously affects their ability to eat.

What is eosinophilic gastritis?

This illness is usually associated with eosinophilic esophagitis and it also involves chronic allergic inflammation, but in the stomach. The main symptoms are nausea and stomach pain.

What is eosinophilic gastroenteritis?

In this illness allergic inflammation occurs all along the gut, and symptoms include pain, poor growth, vomiting, and diarrhea. There can be swelling of the face and body due to protein loss in the gut, leading to protein imbalances. Treatment often requires elimination of multiple foods. As with eosinophilic esophagitis (described more below), it is difficult to identify exactly which foods are problematic in people with eosinophilic gastroenteritis. The natural course of the illness is not well studied.

What are typical symptoms of eosinophilic esophagitis?

The inflammation swells the esophagus, making it hard for it to do its job of squeezing food down to the stomach. Therefore, there is pain with food going down, or the food may not go down at all and get stuck. People with this illness may chew their food for a long time and drink a lot of water with meals to compensate for the problem. When there is vomiting, it may be mucousy and sticky because of the chemicals released from the allergy cells. There can be heartburn symptoms as well. If food gets stuck going down, there may be drooling because the esophagus is blocked. This feeling might mimic anaphylaxis. Young children may have poor growth.

What causes eosinophilic esophagitis?

There appears to be an inherited disposition to having inflammation in the esophagus. The usual triggers seem to be allergens.

How common is eosinophilic esophagitis?

This illness appears to affect as many as 1 in 1,000.

Does eosinophilic esophagitis run in families?

Yes.

Who is at risk for eosinophilic esophagitis?

People with food and other allergies or with a history of eosinophilic esophagitis in the family are at risk. The illness is more common in boys.

At what age is eosinophilic esophagitis usually diagnosed?

The typical ages of diagnosis are during childhood or among adults in their 30s and 40s. However, the illness can occur in all age groups, including infants.

How is eosinophilic esophagitis diagnosed?

Symptoms of vomiting, pain, reflux (heartburn), and especially food getting stuck going down may raise suspicion. A biopsy, performed by putting a tube down the esophagus, is the only way to test for this disease or whether it is responding to therapies.

Are biopsies dangerous?

No. After the person is asleep from the medications, a tube with a camera (endoscope) is put down the esophagus. The esophagus is inspected for signs of inflammation (like a rash) and small "bites" of the surface are taken for checking under a microscope. The procedure is generally over in about 20 minutes, and the risks are minimal (anesthesia risks and risk of bleeding or tearing the esophagus, which are extremely uncommon).

What role does food allergy play in eosinophilic esophagitis?

In studies of children, food is usually shown to be a trigger. For some people, allergens in the air, such as pollens, are important causes, and for others, the inflammation has no obvious trigger. In adults, the relationship between foods and eosinophilic esophagitis has not been tested as thoroughly, but foods probably play a role.

Can removal of food allergens improve eosinophilic esophagitis?

Yes, but often many foods are triggers.

How do you determine which foods are triggering eosinophilic esophagitis?

Suspicions about food triggers are addressed based on personal history, knowledge about common food triggers, testing, elimination diets, food challenges, and biopsies. The primary way to determine if a particular food is a trigger is to remove it from the diet and then perform a biopsy to see if the inflammation improved. Or, if inflammation was under control after some dietary changes were made, another biopsy could be performed after a food was introduced to see if it was tolerated or if it triggered inflammation. This is a tedious process because multiple foods might be triggers.

What are the common food triggers for eosinophilic esophagitis?

The major allergens that cause sudden allergic reactions are triggers, especially milk but also eggs, wheat, soy, peanuts, tree nuts, fish, and shellfish. Triggers for eosinophilic esophagitis also include corn, beef, and many others.

What role do allergy tests play in diagnosing food allergies in eosinophilic esophagitis?

Only a minimal one. Although allergy tests are often performed, they do not correlate well with identifying the true triggers, so trials of dietary avoidance are usually needed. Allergy blood tests, prick skin tests, and even patch tests (see chapter 3) might be used, but none have proven reliability for this illness. They may be used as guides.

How important are elimination diets and feeding tests in diagnosing eosinophilic esophagitis?

Eliminating targeted foods to watch for resolution of symptoms and improvement in biopsies as well as food challenges followed by biopsies and observation are the main approaches to diagnosing food triggers in eosinophilic esophagitis. There are many possible approaches, such as removing one or many foods and waiting for a response over subsequent weeks; making a diet that includes only a list of foods that are probably safe based on the person's history and test results; or using a diet that relies on the nonallergenic amino acid–based formula.

How are medications used to treat eosinophilic esophagitis?

The most effective therapy currently is steroids. Giving regular doses of steroids—for example, by giving pills or injections —carries side effects. Current treatment is aimed at trying to coat the esophagus with steroids, similar to putting a cream on a rash. The person swallows a form of steroids usually used in asthma inhalers.

Should diet changes or medications be used to treat eosinophilic esophagitis?

This is often based on personal preference and trial and error, seeing what works better and what is less stressful to do. Often, a combination approach is needed.

What are the risks of diet treatment of eosinophilic esophagitis?

The diet may be very limited, carrying social and nutritional consequences. Rarely, a food removed from the diet may trigger a sudden allergic reaction when reintroduced. A dietitian may be needed to provide nutritional advice if many foods are eliminated.

What are the risks of medical treatment of eosinophilic esophagitis?

The steroids can cause localized dryness and an increased risk of fungal infection in the esophagus. In small doses, the medication should not affect growth, but growth monitoring is recommended for children.

Why does eosinophilic esophagitis need to be treated?

Two reasons. First, the illness is very uncomfortable, and treatment should address the symptoms. Second, if the inflammation is left unchecked, there could be scarring.

How serious is the risk of scarring in eosinophilic esophagitis?

Some persons with this illness develop scarring that constricts the esophagus, and they require a procedure that stretches the tube to let food down, a procedure that may need to be performed periodically. Biopsies may detect scarring early, but we do not yet know who gets scarring, how fast it happens, and whether treating it early totally reverses it. This situation is frustrating, when treatment improves symptoms but leaves some degree of inflammation. It is not totally clear if the inflammation and scarring may also increase the risk of cancer of the esophagus.

How does one know when eosinophilic esophagitis is being treated properly?

When symptoms are improved and a biopsy shows that the inflammation is resolved or substantially lessened.

Will eosinophilic esophagitis go away?

This illness appears to be persistent and chronic for most people affected.

Besides diet and steroids, are there other treatments on the horizon?

Active research is looking at treatments that might better reduce the inflammation, such as injected antibodies that disable eosinophils, the main problem in this illness. Other antiallergy treatments, such as antihistamines, and medications called cromolyn and antileukotrienes have been evaluated without significant success. There is also research into ways to better diagnose without having to do biopsies. See chapter 10 for more information on future treatments.

Is eosinophilic esophagitis treatable with anti-reflux medications?

A trial of stomach acid–blocking medications is recommended because sometimes this treatment is all that is needed to reverse the inflammation.

Delving Deeper:
DELAYED ALLERGIC REACTIONS

Why are there delayed reactions to some foods?
Delayed and chronic allergic reactions to foods are a result of immune cells causing inflammation, rather than IgE antibodies causing sudden release of chemicals that trigger hives and anaphylaxis. For FPIES, we think that cells called T-cells release chemicals that cause the symptoms. For eosinophilic esophagitis, we think that cells put out chemicals that "call" the troublemakers, the eosinophils, into the esophagus. For atopic dermatitis (eczema), we think that immune cells release various chemicals that bring additional cells into the skin, causing symptoms.

Also of Interest:
CHRONIC ILLNESSES THAT ARE NOT RELATED TO FOOD ALLERGIES

Why do some people say that chronic problems like autism, epilepsy, headaches, arthritis, and hyperactivity are caused by food allergies?
There are theories that foods play a role in many illnesses, and people often use the term "allergy" when talking about this connection. The word "allergy" actually refers to immune responses, so most of the theories should not be using the term "food allergy." Some theories hold that chemicals in milk or wheat play a role in autism, but I am not aware of any studies that confirm this relationship, and scientists have mostly concluded there is no clear relationship. Studies are ongoing to evaluate the role of diet in autism. Nonetheless, there does not appear to be an allergy involved, not even in the theories as described.

Epilepsy (seizures) treatment has been approached with removal of allergens from the diet without clear effect or clear reasoning to support the approach. Some types of seizure disorders, however, respond to a special type of "starvation" diet, which has nothing to do with allergies. Regarding headaches, it is thought that some dietary components, especially tyramine or similar chemicals and perhaps natural histamines, found in foods such as wines, banana, cheeses, bouillon, soy sauce, pickled herring, chocolate, and canned meats, are able to trigger migraines in some sensitive persons. Some literature links rheumatoid arthritis flares to foods. The relationship is unproved, but if it does exist, it may have to do with the inflammatory aspects of the foods, such as a lack of healthful fatty acids. Regarding behavioral problems, childhood hyperactivity has been related to chemical food additives in some children. These issues are discussed in chapter 1 as well.

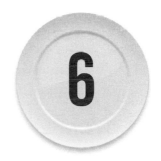

How Do I
AVOID ALLERGIC
REACTIONS to Foods?

In this chapter, I answer questions about avoiding allergic reactions and managing food allergies at home, when shopping, when dining out, in school, at camps, at work, when traveling, and in other settings.

GENERAL QUESTIONS ABOUT AVOIDING ALLERGIC REACTIONS

What do I need to know to keep myself and others safe from food allergens?
It is necessary to think about allergen avoidance at every meal and social circumstance. Knowledge about cross-contact and label reading is key. You may feel overwhelmed by everything you need to know, but reading this chapter should help. Accidents can happen, but being prepared and educated can go a long way in maintaining safety.

What are some common mistakes people make when avoiding a food allergen?
Accidental exposures to avoided allergens often occur when people drop their guard, not thinking about or assuming the safety of a food. Constant vigilance is needed to consider the safety of foods at each meal and snack. Ingredient labels must be read carefully. When food is offered by others, they must understand about food allergies and how to create a "safe" meal.

Mistakes also occur from failure to recognize cross-contact of allergens into otherwise safe foods.

How do I avoid the common mistakes in avoiding food allergens?

Educate yourself and others and always stay vigilant!

If I am curious whether my or my child's allergy has resolved, is it all right to try a small amount of the food?

NO! Always talk to your allergist if you are curious or suspect an allergy has waned or resolved. Testing and possibly a doctor-supervised feeding test may be warranted, but do not try this at home.

Is it a good strategy to assess the safety of a food with a small bite, checking for mouth itch?

This is a potentially dangerous approach sometimes wrongly used to by-pass asking meaningful questions about ingredients and food preparation. The strategy is faulty because often there is no mouth itch prior to having a severe reaction. A taste test is also unreliable because if there is an allergen in part of a food or meal, the initial bite might not contain it. Additionally, the small taste may not evoke a symptom, but a larger amount, when eaten, could. If any antihistamines are being used to treat allergies, these would also reduce or eliminate any mouth symptoms. For all of these reasons, never use this approach to assess the safety of a meal or food.

Is it possible to use a laboratory or test kit to check if a food has an allergen?

Some commercial laboratory tests and some "quick tests" (designed like a pregnancy urine test) detect specific food proteins, such as those in peanuts. Commercial manufacturers might use these tests to check if they have sufficiently cleaned their equipment between running an allergen-containing and an allergen-free product. I do not recommend that individuals use these types of tests, however, to assess, for example, a restaurant meal. Only a small bit of the food is tested, and the allergen could be in some other part of the food. I think it is much safer to ask good questions, follow recommended ways to obtain safe foods, and check product ingredient labels carefully, as described below.

CROSS-CONTACT

What is cross-contact?

Cross-contact, sometimes called cross-contamination, happens when an otherwise allergen-safe food contains an unintentional allergen because of an error during cooking or preparing the food.

What are common examples of allergen cross-contact?

- Using the same knife in peanut butter and then putting it into the jelly jar. Now the jelly jar has some peanut in it that may be introduced into an otherwise safe jelly sandwich at another time.

- A spatula used to loosen some nut-containing cookies from a pan is then used to serve nut-free cookies, introducing nuts onto those cookies.

- French fries are made in a fryer that cooked fried shrimp and fish sticks. Now the French fries have fish and shellfish proteins on them.

- A hamburger is fried on a skillet where a cheeseburger was just cooked, introducing milk onto the hamburger.

- A shake mixer is used to make a peanut-flavored milkshake. A peanut-free milkshake is now blended with the same mixer that was not cleaned, introducing peanut into the peanut-free milkshake.

- A wok used for cashew chicken is now used to heat beef and broccoli, introducing nut proteins into that dish.

- Nuts are chopped on a cutting board that is next used to chop lettuce for a nut-free salad, introducing nut proteins into the salad.

- A mixing spoon used to stir cream soup is next used to stir vegetable soup, introducing milk into the milk-free soup.

- A food handler does not change gloves as she touches a food allergen and then handles food that was intended to be allergen-free.

How does one avoid cross-contact?

There has to be an ongoing consciousness about cross-contact to maintain a safe supply of allergen-free ingredients for meals. This may be possible in a home where family members know that they need to take care to keep ingredients allergen-free at all times. It may be unlikely to occur in places where there is not a constant need to maintain an allergen-free source of ingredients, such as in restaurants, bakeries, or homes without allergic individuals. Therefore, depending on the circumstances, there may be a need for ongoing vigilance (at home) or for education on how to make individual meals that are allergen-safe (for restaurants, friends' homes, and so on).

In an ice cream shop, is washing the scoop sufficient to avoid an allergen?

No. If the scoop was previously used in several ice cream containers, there could already be cross-contact of allergens in the ice cream tubs. For example, if the patron before you ordered a double scoop of vanilla and peanut, the peanut might already have been spread into the vanilla. A clean scoop used in the vanilla would not alter the contamination.

What are some tips to avoid cross-contact with allergens?

Keep foods covered in cupboards and refrigerators. Make the safe food for the person with allergies and set it aside before making foods that contain the allergen. Teach others to avoid the pitfalls described above.

AMOUNTS THAT TRIGGER A REACTION AND CASUAL EXPOSURE

How much food needs to be eaten to trigger a reaction?

The amount of food that can trigger a reaction depends on an individual's sensitivity. It is not easily predicted by any simple tests. For some people, trace amounts that are not easily visible to the naked eye may cause symptoms and for others, a meal-size amount of a food or more may be required to trigger a reaction. Your doctor may be able to assess your level of sensitivity based on your history or your response to a feeding test.

Can smelling a food cause an allergic reaction?
Yes, but this type of exposure is unlikely to cause anaphylaxis.

When can smelling a food cause an allergic reaction?
When the protein from the food is distributed into the air.

Under what circumstances would food proteins become airborne?
This most often occurs from heating, such as in cooking. For example, the steam from scrambling eggs or frying fish and the vapor from boiling or frothing milk can carry proteins into the air. Another way proteins can get into the air is when the food is in a powdery form and gets disturbed, for example, when preparing foods with wheat flour, powdered milk, or dried egg powder. Last, manipulations of a food might spread some proteins into the air nearby, for example, when peeling an orange or cracking peanuts.

In what settings might there be an abundance of food proteins in the air?
Examples include occupational settings, such as a bakery or food-processing factory; markets where a high concentration of the food is being processed or heated, such as a seafood market; food stands or kitchen locations where foods are being heated, such as roasting nuts, or frothing milk at a coffee shop.

Is smelling a food likely to cause an allergic reaction?
Rarely. Most smells from foods are due to organic compounds and no appreciable proteins. For example, the smell of peanut butter is not from any significant protein in the air. Odors from foods that are not being actively heated are unlikely to expel any appreciable allergenic proteins.

What kinds of symptoms might happen from airborne food proteins?
The symptoms would be similar to those from allergens such as pollens and animal danders. Namely, there may be itchy eyes, sneezing, runny nose, and for people with asthma, a cough or wheeze.

Can touching a food cause an allergic reaction?
Yes, but anaphylaxis is unlikely.

What kinds of symptoms might happen from touching a food?
The most common skin symptoms are red blotches, hives, and itchiness. But touching the food does not usually cause symptoms. The skin barrier prevents the proteins from reaching the immune system. Younger children are often more susceptible to skin reactions from direct contact, especially if their skin barrier is compromised by eczema rashes. The eyes are also sensitive to allergens, so an allergen from the fingers rubbed into the eyes can result in significant redness and swelling.

Can a severe reaction happen from touching or smelling a food?
Rarely. If a person with asthma breathes in a large inhalation of a food allergen, a significant asthma attack might occur. If a large area of abraded skin is exposed to an allergen, there may be more absorption, leading to stronger reactions. However, these are unusual circumstances. The primary concern about casual exposure to a food is transferring the food from fingers into the mouth.

What are some surprising mistakes that have led to allergic reactions?
Our studies showed that sometimes parents or other family members fed an allergen purposefully to a child with allergies, or allergic individuals purposefully ate foods they were allergic to, resulting in reactions. The reasons for this include curiosity, thinking a small amount would be ok, and testing to see if the allergy had resolved. If you are unsure you have an allergy, always discuss this with your doctor before trying an allergen at home. Teach caretakers the same.

Is it okay for a person with egg allergy to color Easter eggs?
Yes, but carefully. The most potent part of egg is the white, and raw egg is the most potent form of egg allergen. Sometimes the surface of the egg has the egg white on it, and if the eggs break, there will be an even larger exposure. The skin contact isn't likely to trigger a significant reaction, but doing a craft project with the eggs and then rubbing egg-white-laden fingers into the eye could induce swelling. Participation might include using plastic eggs, wearing gloves, or being careful not to place your fingers in your eyes or mouth.

Can a person with tree nut allergy be near oak trees with acorns?

Acorns are tree nuts, and they might be allergens if eaten, but they are too sour to eat, so there is no literature about reactions from eating them. Like other nuts, it is not likely that touching them would result in any significant allergic reactions.

Can a person with seafood allergy swim in the ocean?

Yes. I am not aware of any reports of a person being allergic to seawater based on an allergy to fish or shellfish. This is probably true for several reasons. The dilution of proteins in the ocean is tremendous. The concentration of allergenic protein in the water becomes irrelevant. Second, the allergenic proteins in fish or shellfish are muscle proteins that would not be directly leaching into the water.

Can a person with a fish allergy own pet fish?

Yes, since the allergenic proteins are inside the fish and are not being eaten. However, the fish food is often made of fish and shellfish. If you are handling the food, minimize skin exposure by tapping the food into the water from a cap or container and washing your hands afterward. The main risk here might be rubbing the fish food on your hand into the eye, causing swelling.

Can a person with a fish allergy go fishing?

Yes, although handling the fish or handling parts of the fish after cleaning could irritate the skin because of localized allergic reactions. The main risk would be of skin or eye reactions, and possibly ingestion reactions if there is transfer to the mouth. It is possible to enjoy fishing by reducing direct handling of the fish, rinsing hands afterwards, and wearing gloves when possible.

Can a person with a seafood allergy go to a dolphin show or swim with dolphins?

Dolphins themselves do not have allergenic fish proteins because they are mammals, but they are fed fish and swim in an enclosed area where dilution is less than that seen in the ocean. Therefore, there is some risk that the fish proteins they ingest are in the pool water and may cause symptoms for a person with a fish allergy. I have had patients develop hives from the water when splashed at shows.

Can a person with a food allergy swim in a pool with others who may have eaten the food?

When young children are snacking and swimming, there is some risk that they may share food, so supervision is needed. A better choice is not to eat while swimming. There is a risk of choking as well! The small amount of residual allergens that might be in a mouth or on the body of a person who is swimming is unlikely to be relevant to the allergic swimmer because of the dilution effect of the pool. This risk might increase if people are constantly eating in the pool and spilling food and if the pool is small. However, in most situations, there should be no significant concern about reacting to residual food proteins in a swimming pool.

Can a person be allergic to seawater, pool water, or any water?

Yes, but usually this is caused by the temperature of the water. There is a problem called cold urticaria, where swimming in cold water, or coming out of a pool and getting chilled, causes hives. This is a kind of physically induced reaction where, we believe, the allergy cells respond to the change in temperature. It is rare for this form of reaction to progress beyond the skin. Antihistamines are often used for treatment. There is another rare illness, called aquagenic urticaria, where water of any temperature on the skin causes hives, but the person can still drink water.

Can tiny shrimp, copepods, in drinking water cause an allergic reaction?

Get ready to become a little grossed out. Yes, there is a microscopic animal related to shrimp that lives in freshwater and is allowed to remain in safe drinking water, especially from sources in geographic areas that have excellent natural water available for drinking. When sources of natural drinking water exceed government standards, the water is unfiltered, leaving these microscopic animals behind. No harmful effects have been related to these creatures. Presumably if they have shellfish-relevant proteins, there is too little to trigger a reaction based on the small size and dilution effects of the otherwise safe and clean drinking water. Thus, they seem not to be a concern. If you are concerned, a home water filter could remove them.

If a cow, pig, or chicken is fed allergens such as peanut or soy, can I be allergic to that animal's meat?

This should not be a concern because the animal's meat proteins do not change based on its diet. It does not have these food proteins within its meat.

Can a person with a food allergy go shopping in a supermarket?

Although every allergen is in the store, it is not likely that allergic reactions would be elicited merely from shopping. Still, there are a few things to consider. Before seating an allergic toddler in a shopping cart, it is prudent to wipe the surfaces since it is likely that the child might suck on the handle bar or other surfaces. If there is a shellfish allergy, it may be prudent to avoid the area where seafood is being steamed as this might force the seafood proteins into the air transiently.

AVOIDANCE AT HOME

Does a food allergen need to be removed entirely from the home?

Usually not, but personal preferences and the ages and diets of the household members may dictate your decision. For example, if there is a person with peanut allergy in the household, and no other family member insists on eating this food, it may be easier to exclude peanut from the home since it is not a common ingredient in most foods. Conversely, most households do not restrict foods such as milk or egg because they are common components in the diet. If there are many young children with food allergies in a home, it may be easier to exclude certain ingredients to reduce the risk of unintentional sharing among the siblings. Overall, there are many options as long as care is taken for food storage, preparation, and supervision during meals.

What do people do to stay safe when they allow a food allergen in the home?
There have to be precautions in place to reduce cross-contact, keep unsafe foods away from young children who cannot self-monitor, and stay organized about knowing which foods are safe.

What are some tips for maintaining a safe home that allows the food allergen?
Consider the following:

- Teach all family members about cross-contact and not sharing food.
- Prepare the allergen-safe meal ahead of those containing the allergen.
- Specify certain shelves for allergen-safe foods in cupboards or refrigerators.
- Specify counter areas as "allergen-safe" for preparation of foods for the person with a food allergy.
- Use color-coding labels on purchased products and storage containers, such as green for safe and red for allergens.
- Supervise young, food-allergic children during mealtimes to prevent sharing.
- Keep allergenic foods out of reach of young, food-allergic children.
- Clean dishware and utensils appropriately.

Does the heat of a skillet, griddle, or fryer destroy allergens?
No.

What type of cleaning is needed to remove food allergens from dishes and utensils?
Normal cleaning with soap and water should be sufficient.

Does a standard dishwasher adequately remove allergens from dishes and utensils?
Dishwashers are reliable. However, be sure to rinse off any solid food buildup before washing. If the dishware and utensils appear clean after washing, without evident residue, the cleaning process is almost certainly appropriate to have removed allergens.

Is it safe to cook allergen-safe foods in ovens and microwaves where allergens were cooked?

If the allergens were heated at another time, and the safe food is in a dish so that it is not in contact with the oven surfaces, there should be no problem. If the allergen is being heated in an open container along with another open container that has safe foods at the same time, there is a risk that the allergen may splatter or that steam from the allergen may land in the safe food. Heating the foods separately or covered should allay such problems.

Is it safe to cook allergen-safe foods on grills where allergens were cooked?

If the grill is not specifically cleaned, there could be residual allergens. The heat of the grill may not destroy them. One option is to heat the allergen-safe food on aluminum foil on the grill.

PURCHASING MANUFACTURED PRODUCTS

What can I learn from reading a product label?

Except under unusual circumstances, the label should list all ingredients. This usually allows identification of any allergens. Surprisingly, however, some products have hidden ingredients that are not fully disclosed.

Do I need to read labels every time?

Yes. Ingredients can change, so reading the label each time ensures that you are aware of any new ingredients that could be problematic.

Is it helpful to develop a list of "safe products"?

No, it can be a dangerous practice. Often families, schools, or organizations wish to create lists of products that are safe for an individual so that the labels do not need to be read each time. However, ingredients change, so the list can become outdated right away. It is better practice to read the label each time.

Can ingredients vary in the same product from time to time?

Yes. Sometimes different sizes of the same product have slightly different ingredients. Sometimes a product made in one location differs somewhat from the same product manufactured in another factory. By reading the label each time, you can avoid unpleasant surprises from unexpected ingredients.

What do the U.S. food allergen–labeling laws require?

The Food Allergen Labeling and Consumer Protection Act of 2004 (FALCPA) requires that major allergens—milk, eggs, wheat, soy, peanuts, tree nuts, fish, and crustacean shellfish—that are intended ingredients in a food be listed in plain English somewhere on the ingredient label. The law applies to all packaged foods regulated under the Federal Food, Drug, and Cosmetic Act (FFD&C Act). Also, the type of nut (for example, walnut, almond) and species of fish (such as bass, tuna) or crustacean shellfish (such as lobster, shrimp) must be named specifically. There are various options for declaring the allergen; for example, the ingredient list might say "milk" or it might show the allergen in parentheses—"whey (milk)"—or there might be a separate line noting, "Contains milk." Highly processed, refined oils that are essentially free from proteins are exempt from labeling laws.

Do the U.S. labeling laws apply to imported foods?

Yes, they apply to domestic and imported foods. There is a system in place to check the labeling as the shipment enters the country, and the labels can be revised, if needed. This system does not actually "test" products to verify ingredients. It just ensures that the labeling practices are following U.S. laws.

What do the FDA and the labeling laws consider to be nuts?

Many: almond, beechnut, Brazil, butternut, cashew, chestnut, chinquapin, coconut, filbert / hazelnut, ginkgo, hickory nut, lychee nut, macadamia nut (bush nut), pecan, pine nut / piñon, pili nut, pistachio, shea nut, walnut (heartnut).

What is not covered by the U.S. labeling laws?

Any food that is not considered a major allergen, including seeds, spices, and non-crustacean seafood, such as clams and squid. Also, the laws do not currently mandate the labeling that warns of possible contamination with allergens (advisory or precautionary labeling). Meat, poultry, and egg products and other "raw" agricultural foods (fruits, vegetables, and so on) are not covered. Cosmetics and medications are not part of the laws, although allergens are often declared. Alcoholic beverages may contain allergens, including unexpected ones such as eggs, cow's milk, or seafood (used as clarifying agents). FALCPA does not cover alcoholic beverages, although the federal agency that oversees labeling of alcohol has stated an intention to apply similar rules in the near future. The relevance of allergens used as clarifying agents in wine is mostly unknown, but a couple of studies indicate no significant risk.

What is a "free from" statement?

Some manufacturers voluntarily label a product "free from" an allergen. They presumably do this to indicate that there is no risk of contamination, and they may be directing their product to persons with a food allergy. However, there are no laws regarding this type of labeling.

What is a "contains" statement?

This is a separate statement, usually near the ingredients list, that discloses the major allergens in the food. This type of labeling is an option.

Can a "contains" statement show only the names of major food allergen sources that are not already identified in the ingredients list?

No. If a "contains" statement is used on a food label, it is supposed to include the names of the food sources of all major food allergens used as ingredients in the food. For example, if "whey," "egg yolks," and "natural peanut flavor" are declared in a product's ingredients list, the "contains" statement is required to identify all three sources of the major food allergens present ("Contains milk, eggs, peanuts"), not just some of them.

Will the ingredients label identify each and every ingredient?
No, the label may hide some proprietary ingredients under collective labels, such as "natural flavors" or "spices." This is not the case for the major allergens included in the labeling laws.

Is there any way to find out what ingredients are in a food with ambiguous labeling such as "spices"?
It depends on the willingness of the manufacturer. I suggest that if you are interested in buying the product, you may want to pose your question in a way that does not require a full "secret" ingredient disclosure. For example, you might say, "I am allergic to sesame. Is there any sesame in the spices or flavorings in your product?" If you had an allergic reaction to a food and aren't sure what caused the reaction, you should work with your doctor to get more information from the manufacturer, because it is important to track down the allergen to prevent future reactions.

What are advisory or precautionary statements?
These are voluntary statements that indicate a possible risk that an allergen could be unintentionally included in the food. There are no laws requiring these statements or guidelines on how to describe the concern, but the statements must be truthful. Manufacturers state this possibility in many different ways: "may contain ____," "in a facility that processes ____," "made on equipment with ____," "processed in a facility that also processes ____," and many others.

Do the words used in advisory statements differentiate the degree of risk?
No. You might assume that "May contain peanuts" is riskier than "in a facility that also processes peanuts," but this is not the case.

How often does the product with an advisory label have the allergen in it?
Our studies have shown the risk to be in the range of about 2% to 10%, but this varies by allergen and types of food. For example, there was a high rate of milk found in chocolate products that did not have intentional milk ingredients. Additionally, there is variation from time to time and batch to batch.

How much of the allergen might be in a product with an advisory label?
As an unintended ingredient, the amounts are typically low, but there may be enough to trigger reactions in sensitive people. Most allergists will advise avoidance of these products, but you should discuss this with your allergist in case you are not very sensitive and don't need to be as concerned.

If a product does not have an advisory label, does that mean there is no risk?
Technically, no. Since advisory labeling is voluntary, an unintended ingredient could be in a food without a warning.

How often would a product without an advisory warning contain an allergen?
In our studies of products we suspected of this (such as a baked good), we found this type of error uncommon but more likely to occur with smaller companies (a few products we tested for milk or egg had trace amounts). However, among 120 products that did not mention peanuts on the label, none had detectable peanut.

Do I need to call manufacturers of every product to ask them if their food could be contaminated with an allergen?
It is difficult to recommend this degree of burdensome checking. As indicated above, the risks are generally low, and larger manufacturers (Kraft, General Mills, and so on) can generally be trusted. Caution about smaller companies, especially for baked goods, may be advisable.

Will the food allergy labeling laws change?
They may, either to include more foods or to alter some of the regulations. You can check for updates at the FDA's website: www.fda.gov/Food/FoodSafety/FoodAllergens.

What do I do if I have an allergic reaction to a product and I do not know why?
You should try to keep the package and call the company and your allergist. You may have discovered a problem, such as an unintentional contamination with an allergen that could lead to a recall, or you may have an allergy to an ingredient you did not know about. You can contact

the complaint center in your area at www.fda.gov/opacom/backgrounders /complain.html. You can also contact the FDA's Center for Food Safety and Applied Nutrition Adverse Event Reporting System by phone at (301) 436–2405, by email at CAERS@cfsan.fda.gov, or by mail at FDA, CAERS, HFS-700, 2A-012/CPK1, 5100 Paint Branch Parkway, College Park, MD 20740.

What should I know about labeling laws in other countries?

Labeling laws vary among countries (and some have none). Many nations have laws that include more than just the major eight foods currently covered by the U.S. laws. For example, the European Union enacted legislation in 2005 requiring that the following allergens, not covered in U.S. laws, be listed: rye, barley, oats, celery, mustard, and sesame seeds. Canada requires labeling that is similar to the United States but adds sesame and mustard. Research ahead of your trip to understand the laws where you are traveling.

How would I know if a mistake had been made in a food label?

Rarely, a food label will have an error, or a food allergen will have been added by mistake without labeling. Such foods, when identified, are recalled. You can get on a mailing list regarding food recalls for allergen-labeling errors at www.foodallergy.org.

RESTAURANTS

Do restaurants know what to do for a person with food allergies?

Some may, but you should make no assumptions. Always discuss your allergy very carefully with restaurant personnel.

Will the menu direct me to safe foods?

Some may, but you should never depend on a menu description to identify a safe meal. It is always possible that different ingredients are used than listed, that the list does not include all ingredients, or that the dish has unintended ingredients. Sometimes a food has been prepared ahead of your ordering it and may have ingredients the people in the restaurant do not know about, so always discuss this possibility as well.

What types of mistakes can happen at a restaurant?
The food could have unintended ingredients, hidden or secret ingredients, or an allergen from cross-contact during preparation.

What are examples of hidden ingredients?
- A sauce thickened with peanut flour
- Fish used in a dressing
- Milk used in sauces
- Peanut butter used to seal the ends of an egg roll
- Nuts used in a dressing

How can I alert the restaurant personnel to my allergy?
The best action is to clearly identify that you have an allergy, not just a preference or distaste for a food. Explain that you could get sick if you ate even a small amount of the food you are avoiding. Provide some examples of what can be done wrong that would lead to a problem, as discussed below. Ask to speak with the person responsible for your meal.

With whom should I communicate my needs at a restaurant?
You usually will begin a discussion with a server or manager. Suggest that you would like to speak with whomever is involved with preparing or overseeing the preparation of your meal. Providing some written description of your allergy, for example, a "chef card," may help to emphasize your needs.

Where can I get "chef cards" for restaurant dining?
An example is available at www.foodallergy.org/files/chefcardtemplate .pdf. Foodallergy.org also has a list of resources for chef cards that are free or for sale, including ones in different languages for travel.

Are certain types of restaurants off limits?

Some restaurants may be extremely poor choices, where the risks are too high (depending on the specific allergies). For example, a seafood restaurant is a poor choice for people with fish or shellfish allergies. Asian restaurants, bakeries, and ice cream shops can be a challenge for people with peanut or tree nut allergies. It is not always good enough to ask an ice cream shop to wash the scoop because they may have already contaminated otherwise safe flavors when dipping from container to container. Self-serve buffets can be a challenge since food is often cross-contacted by the patrons. On the other hand, it may be possible to get a safe meal in any of these situations if the staff is understanding and accommodating and if you direct them appropriately.

What are some common pitfalls for people with food allergies eating in restaurants?

- Not explaining clearly that the problem is a true allergy (leading to a poor response)
- The staff making incorrect assumptions, for example, believing that removing an allergen from a finished dish is sufficient
- The staff not realizing an ingredient has allergens in it (milk in butter and egg in mayonnaise)
- Not considering cross-contact during food preparation (shared grills, fryers, blenders, serving utensils, etc.)
- The staff assuming they know the ingredients of a finished food
- Not considering the ingredients of all components of a meal (sauces, garnish)
- Not having medications (always carry your emergency medications)

What are some suggestions to help the restaurant staff provide a safe meal?

Be clear that you have a food allergy, that a small amount of the wrong food could send you to an emergency room or be life threatening. Consider using chef cards that name your allergies and provide hints about allergen avoidance in restaurants. Ask to speak with people who are in charge, especially those who are responsible for the meal preparation, and provide some education as you make your requests by giving some concrete examples. Be specific. My studies on restaurant staff's knowledge showed that sometimes they make assumptions about food allergies that are incorrect (such as thinking that fryer heat destroys allergens).

What can I say to inform restaurant staff about preparing a safe meal?
Consider these examples:

- I am allergic to milk, and any bit of milk or milk products can make me very sick. I want a hamburger, no bun, steamed broccoli, and a baked potato. Please check if the hamburger has any fillers, because they could have milk. I want it cooked on foil on the grill to avoid getting cheese on it from a prior cheeseburger. If the potato or the vegetable looks dry, that is okay, do not put butter on it!

- I am allergic to nuts, and any amount can make me sick. I want the salad without nuts. You cannot just pick the nuts off a premade salad. It has to be made from scratch. And if you chop nuts on a chopping board and then chop my lettuce, the lettuce can have nuts on it and make me sick. I will have the vinaigrette dressing if you can tell me the ingredients, because sometimes they flavor that with nuts. Otherwise, just bring me the oil and the vinegar.

- I am allergic to fish. I know I am just ordering French fries, but if you fry fish in the same oil, I could get sick.

- I am having the turkey sandwich, but I am extremely allergic to milk. Sometimes they flavor turkey with milk, so can you check that? Can I see the package ingredient label for the bread? I will skip it if it has milk. Also, if you slice the turkey on a slicer with cheese, I could get sick. Don't put any dressing on it because that often has milk. I will take ketchup.

What should I do if I think restaurant personnel are not understanding my allergy?
Leave.

What should I do if I get a meal that seems to have my allergen in it?

Hold the meal and ask to see the manager and chef. Sending a meal back could lead to more mistakes (such as having them remove the shrimp and re-serve the same pasta). If you are not comfortable, do not take a chance.

What are some options for going to restaurants with children who have food allergies?

One option is to bring along a safe meal that is similar to what the restaurant serves and explain the situation. It may be helpful to scout out a restaurant without your child first, to discuss what meals they may be able to make safely. Explain that you could become a frequent guest if they can accommodate your needs.

SOCIAL OUTINGS AND FAMILY GATHERINGS

What are some concerns to consider when eating at other people's homes?

Family, friends, and acquaintances are usually not managing their homes day to day with concerns about food allergies. Well-intentioned hosts may not appreciate how to create a safe meal. Large, complex, multi-ingredient meals are associated with various social holidays, such as Christmas and Thanksgiving, as well as with milestone celebrations.

What should be done to obtain safe holiday meals away from home?

Speak with your hosts well in advance. Offer solutions, such as preparing simple, safe meals or bringing safe potluck contributions. Discuss your allergies as you would with a restaurant. Offer to help out in meal preparation. When it is time for the meal, watch young, food-allergic children closely to be sure that they do not take unsafe foods from serving dishes or bowls with treats.

How should I arrange play dates for children with food allergies?

When introducing young children to friends' homes early on, explain your child's allergies and offer to stay for part of the time to explain about emergency medications. Bring safe snacks and discuss alternatives for snack times, or avoid snacks altogether. Be sure that your child, the friends, and supervising adults understand that the play date should be stress-free as long as safe food is eaten and that it should be easy to ensure that this happens. Children without food allergies are often interested in trying the "safe snacks."

Can a child with food allergy go Halloween trick-or-treating?

Yes, but with planning ahead of time. It must be made clear that your child is not to eat any of the treats while out. Provide some safe snacks to bring along. Depending on the child's specific allergies, it may be possible to pick out safe foods based on ingredient labels once you are back home. Alternatively, arrange in advance to trade the bounty for safe treats or activities. For younger children, a few friends could be preselected who have or are provided with some safe treats that can be eaten right away. Never take chances on unlabeled treats!

SCHOOL

What are the main concerns for going to school with food allergies?

The three main concerns are to (1) avoid eating a food allergen, (2) have a plan in place to treat an allergic reaction, especially anaphylaxis, and (3) learn and do everything that the other children are doing except for eating the avoided food.

How do I approach a school about managing my child's food allergies?

Discuss your child's food allergies well in advance. Begin by asking whether the school has other children with food allergies and what the school does to promote safety. I suggest this approach over presenting a large list of "requirements" that the school might view as overwhelming. Determine who coordinates food allergy management for the school. This is usually a school nurse, if there is one. Provide the school with the required documentation about the allergy from your doctor and attain any forms that the school requires in advance. Work with your school, doctor, and child to develop a plan. Ensure that the management plan is communicated with all the individuals who will be supervising your child, including specialty teachers, such as for art, as well as substitute teachers. Discuss how safe meals and snacks will be obtained. Discuss how the emergency plans will be implemented, practiced, and extended to activities outside the school day, such as field trips, special events, and preschool or afterschool activities.

How does school food allergy management differ for various age groups?

The youngest preschool children are more apt to get into trouble by taking unsafe food and placing almost everything in their mouths without concern. These children require strict supervision. Older children may understand not to share foods and can self-manage better. Teenagers should be able to self-manage, including recognizing and treating reactions, but this is also an age group that increases risk taking, and you may not be able to depend on them to self-medicate with epinephrine. Thus, supervision and avoidance strategies change according to age, developmental capabilities, and school resources. I discuss a child's age-related responsibilities later in this chapter.

Is it better to homeschool a child with food allergies to keep him or her safe?

Homeschooling is a fine choice if there is intrinsic interest in this educational approach, but it should not be necessary to homeschool a child solely because of a food allergy.

Are there any guidelines for managing food allergies in schools?

Yes. Some states have guidelines, and national guidelines are emerging. You can usually find your state's guidelines with an Internet search, but here are some examples:

- Massachusetts (www.doe.mass.edu/cnp/allergy.pdf)

- New Jersey (www.state.nj.us/education/students/safety/health/services /allergies.pdf)

- New York (www.health.ny.gov/professionals/protocols_and_guidelines /docs/caring_for_students_with_life_threatening_allergies.pdf)

- Washington (www.foodallergy.org/files/Wash_State_Anaphylaxis
_Guidelines.pdf)

National guidelines are under development and should be available at:
www.cdc.gov/Healthyyouth/foodallergies/index.htm.

What are the responsibilities of families sending their food-allergic children to school?

A family's responsibility can be summarized as follows:

- Notify the school of your child's allergies.

- Work with the school team to develop a plan that accommodates the child's needs throughout the school, including in the classroom, in the cafeteria, in after-care programs, during school-sponsored activities, and on the school bus. Fill out a food allergy action plan (also called an anaphylaxis action plan, food allergy emergency plan, and so forth— see the example in chapter 11) and ensure that everyone has a copy.

- Provide written medical documentation, instructions, and medications as directed by a physician, using the food allergy action plan as a guide. Include a photo of your child on the written form.

- Provide properly labeled medications and replace medications after use or upon expiration.

- Educate your child in food allergy self-management:
  - safe and unsafe foods
  - strategies for avoiding exposure to unsafe foods
  - symptoms of allergic reactions
  - how and when to tell an adult if having an allergy-related problem
  - how to read food labels (age appropriate)

- Review policies and procedures with the school staff, your child's physician, and your child (if age appropriate) after a reaction has occurred.

- Provide emergency contact information.

- Encourage wearing medical identification jewelry.

What are the responsibilities of the school for managing a child's food allergies?
A school's responsibilities may be summarized as follows:

- Be knowledgeable about and follow applicable federal laws, including the Americans with Disabilities Act, Section 504, and any state laws or district policies that apply.

- Review the health records submitted by parents and physicians.

- Include food-allergic students in school activities. Students should not be excluded from school activities solely based on their food allergies.

- Identify a core team of, but not limited to, school nurse, teacher, principal, school food service and nutrition manager, and counselor (if available) to work with parents and the student (age appropriate) to establish a prevention plan. Changes to the prevention plan to promote food allergy management should be made with core team participation.

- Make sure all staff who interact with the student understand food allergy, can recognize symptoms, know what to do in an emergency, and work with other school staff to eliminate the use of food allergens in the allergic student's meals, educational tools, arts and crafts projects, and incentives.

- Practice the food allergy action plans before an allergic reaction occurs to assure the efficiency/effectiveness of the plans.

- Coordinate with the school nurse to be sure medications are appropriately stored, and be sure an emergency kit is available that contains a physician's standing order for epinephrine. In states where regulations permit, medications are kept in an easily accessible secure location central to designated school personnel, not in locked cupboards or drawers.

- Students should be allowed to carry their own epinephrine, if age appropriate, after approval from the student's physician or clinic, parent, and school nurse, as allowed by state or local regulations. See below for more information on this decision.

- Designate school personnel who are properly trained to administer medications in accordance with the State Nursing and Good Samaritan Laws governing the administration of emergency medications.

- Be prepared to handle a reaction and ensure that a staff member is available who is properly trained to administer medications during the school day regardless of time or location.

- Review policies and prevention plans with core team members, parents or guardians, student (age appropriate), and physician after a reaction has occurred.

- Work with the district transportation administrator to make sure school bus driver training includes symptom awareness and what to do if a reaction occurs.

- Recommend that all buses have communication devices in case of an emergency.

- Enforce a "no eating" policy on school buses, with exceptions made only to accommodate special needs under federal or similar laws, or school district policy.

- Discuss appropriate management of food allergy with student families.

- Discuss field trips with the families of food-allergic children to decide appropriate strategies for managing the allergies.

- Follow federal, state, and district laws and regulations regarding sharing medical information about the student.

- Take threats against and harassment or bullying of an allergic child seriously (see chapter 7 for more on bullying).

What are the students' responsibilities for managing food allergies in school?
The students' responsibilities will vary by age and developmental level but may be summarized:

- Should not trade food with others

- Should not eat anything with unknown ingredients or known to contain any allergen

- Should be proactive in the care and management of their food allergies and reactions based on their developmental level

- Should notify an adult immediately if they eat something they believe may contain the food to which they are allergic

What role does hand washing play in food allergen avoidance?

It is presumed that hand washing would reduce finger-to-mouth transfer of allergens should the child with food allergies have touched an allergen. It is presumed that classmates' hand washing after meals would reduce spread of food allergens to materials that are shared by classmates. However, these strategies have not really been tested. Based on what is known about the amounts of foods that might trigger reactions and the low risk of severe reactions from skin exposure, one might expect that hand washing would play a minor role in protecting children with food allergies compared to policies such as not sharing food. The relative benefits may also be influenced by the age of the children, since younger children may be more apt to suck fingers or toys.

Do antibacterial gels and foams remove allergens from hands?

No, just germs. To get allergens off dirty hands requires soap and water or wet wipes.

Do schools or classrooms need to exclude (ban) food allergens?

Banning a food from a specific classroom or a school is one option that is sometimes undertaken to reduce risk. Most often, the ban is applied to peanut and tree nuts. Classroom bans are more common than school-wide ones and are more often aimed at children who are too young to self-monitor. No studies prove that this is an effective strategy, but it is assumed to reduce the risk. However, it remains crucial to enforce the additional strategies listed above to ensure safety. Bans can lead to a false sense of security ("I can share food since nothing has peanut") and to allergic reactions from these false assumptions. Personal issues and the age of the child may come into play in decision making. For example, it may be sensible to "ban" powdery, messy, cheese-puff type snacks from a kindergarten room when one student has a severe milk allergy.

What type of cleaning needs to be done to keep eating areas safe for children with food allergies?

No special chemicals are needed. Soap and water or a wet wipe is typically sufficient to remove allergens. There would need to be some type of physical motion to wipe off the surfaces, not just spread the residue around, even if soap is used.

Can cafeterias provide safe meals for children with food allergies?

Yes, but they must understand how to do so. Talk to your school beforehand to ensure they can successfully avoid the allergens (understand cross-contact, label reading, etc.). Another option is to provide a bagged lunch and snack.

What are some safe food alternatives for children with food allergies in school?

Foods used for craft projects, science experiments, celebrations, and snacks can be substituted. Watch out for unexpected food exposure, such as egg white used to smooth finger paint, or wheat in modeling clays. If foods must be used, consider alternatives such as rice milk for cow's milk. Nonfood treats can be substituted as rewards or for celebrations, for example, birthday pencils or other trinkets. Have safe, nonperishable snacks available for spontaneous celebrations. Talk to the school personnel to be sure that they communicate any special events in advance so that everyone is aware of any issues about food allergy and can address them ahead of time.

What are some alternatives for school celebrations that involve food?

The teacher might instead have a fun activity, such as watching a movie; reading a special book; handing out trinkets, such as birthday pencils, small stuffed animals, or other toys; or adding time to recess instead of having a food celebration. Celebrations could include games with prizes or an arts and crafts project.

How should snack times be managed for children with food allergies?

There are several ways. The responsible adults might ensure that any snack is safe for the entire class; there might be substitute snacks for those with food allergies; or snacks might be limited, with alternative nonfood options for celebrations, such as a celebratory game or toy.

How should lunch and mealtimes be managed for children with food allergies?

It depends on the child's age. Younger children will need more supervision. If there is no allergen-safe table, more supervision to prevent sharing may be needed. The allergic child might be seated toward a table's end and near a supervising adult. It is generally good practice to limit mealtimes to locations designated for them when possible, rather than having young children carry snacks or food throughout play areas, where the allergic child might take them. If the meal is eaten at a table that can be cleaned afterward and then used for any other activities, there is less chance that foods of danger to the young child will be left in reach. I am not in favor of having a child sit alone or separated. If there is a medical need to keep the child away from others eating the allergen, which would be quite unusual, then options such as inviting some friends who are eating safe foods to eat with the child who has allergies is an option. Older children who are not likely to take unsafe foods from others would usually require much less supervision or concern.

Do we need an allergen-free table or cafeteria?

I prefer the term "allergen-safe" table or cafeteria when there are instructions to have a food, such as peanuts or nuts, banned. Whether you believe your child needs this type of accommodation would require consideration of your child's age and ability to understand not taking another child's food, as well as of particular circumstances of the allergy and school setting described previously. My bias is that the majority of children with food allergies who know not to take another's food should not need special seating arrangements. The options should be discussed with your allergist and school.

Why do you prefer the term "allergen-safe" rather than "allergen-free"?

This is to avoid the notion that food sharing would be acceptable if allergens were banned. In reality, people who are not living with food allergies on a daily basis may not be sending "safe" foods to school. There could be a false sense of security. I am aware of reactions in "peanut-free" settings because of this circumstance.

How should preschool time and afterschool activities and sports be managed for children with food allergies?

Ensure that all of the adults who are supervising a child with food allergies are aware of the allergies. Otherwise, unsafe foods might be offered, reactions unnoticed, and emergency plans not arranged properly.

Does a child with food allergies need a paraprofessional to maintain safety in the school setting?

A "para" is an individual assigned to provide individualized attention to a child, in this case to assist the child in avoiding the food and recognizing or initiating treatment of an allergic reaction. The decision to request or grant this level of service is individualized according to the child, the allergies, and the school circumstances. In my experience, the need for this is exceptional because there are many options for successful avoidance.

What should be done about bus transportation for children with food allergies?

Ideally, the bus driver would be able to take responsibility for a child's food allergy just as a teacher does. Local regulations, however, may prevent the driver from taking on the full responsibilities of an emergency action plan. Good Samaritan laws would still apply in an emergency.

What are the key issues to address regarding bus transportation for a child with food allergies?

- Ensure that the driver is informed about your child's allergies, symptoms, and requirements for treatment in the event of an allergic reaction.

- Request no eating on the bus, no food parties.

- Have the younger children with food allergies sit at the front of the bus under improved supervision of the driver.

- Insist that the driver have a communication device, such as a cell phone, and discuss emergency procedures, such as calling 911 and providing the necessary details in the event of an emergency on the bus (this would include not only allergy but also any other general emergencies, such as a bus accident, or medical emergencies, such as seizures or injuries).

Should there be epinephrine on the bus?

Ideally, self-injectable epinephrine would be onboard, although sometimes circumstances and regulations prevent this option. The child may be allowed to self-carry, although depending on the child to self-inject is not usually reasonable. See later in this chapter for more discussion on these topics.

What can be done to reduce the risk of a food-allergic reaction on the bus?

The risk of having an allergic reaction on the school bus is minimized by ensuring a safe meal and no symptoms prior to boarding. The most serious error I have seen was a school placing a child on a bus during an allergic reaction with the misguided notion that the child would best be managed by the parent upon arrival at home. The degree of concern and special accommodations might vary according to your child's age, developmental ability, and specific allergies, but most children with food allergies are able to ride the school bus safely with the minimal accommodations described above. Concerns about significant reactions from residual, invisible food proteins on seats are not typically warranted, but a seat could be wet-wiped if needed for a young child.

How should field trips be managed for children with food allergies?

Remind the school about extending food allergy management to activities outside the school building. Parents should be informed about field trips in advance. Decisions may need to be made about avoiding high-risk activities, for example touring a peanut factory for a child with peanut allergy. Safe meals would need to be arranged in advance, such as a bagged lunch, and an adult able to recognize and treat allergic reactions should be available.

What emergency plans should be in place in the event of an allergic reaction at school?

Individuals supervising your child should be educated about the allergy, recognition of symptoms, and how to activate an emergency response, such as giving epinephrine promptly. In some cases, this would mean that the supervising adult provides treatment, but in most cases, it means alerting the on-site health care professional or that person's delegate. The emergency plan typically includes providing medications according to symptoms, activating emergency services by calling 911, and then informing parents.

Who is responsible for the emergency plans in a school?

Typically the school nurse is responsible for the details of the emergency plans and educating others about the allergy and treatment response, including when and how to use epinephrine. Otherwise, it may be necessary to work through school administration.

What are the differences in management for schools with and without a school nurse?

When there is no on-site school nurse, delegates would be required to understand how to recognize and manage food allergies. Even with a nurse, this is good policy, so that others in the school are able to provide backup. Often the principal and vice principal would take primary responsibility, but additional teachers may be part of the management team. When there is an on-site school nurse, it is often preferable to alert that person to manage an allergic reaction. There would typically not be much time lost in alerting a school nurse through an intercom system, but having backup delegates available in case of delay is prudent.

Does every child in a school require his or her own emergency plan and medications?

Yes, although new laws may allow a general prescription of and administration of epinephrine to children who do not have a prior anaphylaxis diagnosis or emergency plan.

What key points should be addressed for emergency management of an allergic reaction in school?

- There should be a written action plan that the supervising adults are familiar with.

- There should be a procedure in place for activation of the plan in the event of an emergency, such as a strategy to promptly inform the nurse or delegate.

- Procedures for obtaining and administering emergency medications should be well-known and rehearsed.

- Procedures for activating emergency services and communicating with parents should be rehearsed.

- Emergency plans should be considered in the context of special circumstances, such as field trips, special activities, and emergencies such as a lockdown.

Where should epinephrine be stored?

Ideally, in a widely known, unlocked location with prompt access. Depending on the school's physical layout, this may entail a location in or near a cafeteria, in the administration's office, or in the nursing office.

How many doses of epinephrine should be available?

At least two doses should be accessible.

Should a student carry emergency medications?

When the student is capable of self-carrying and self-treatment, and local guidelines allow it, this is a reasonable approach, especially if the medication would not be accessible within a few minutes.

How does one know when a student is capable of carrying emergency medications?

Here are some considerations:

For students

- They express a desire to carry and self-administer epinephrine
- They are deemed of appropriate age, maturity, or developmental level
- They can identify signs and symptoms of anaphylaxis
- They can demonstrate knowledge of proper medication use in response to signs and symptoms
- They demonstrate correct technique in administering epinephrine (with a trainer)
- They are willing to comply with school's rules about use of medicine at school, for example:
  - Keeping the autoinjector of epinephrine with them at all times
  - Notifying a responsible adult (for example, teacher, nurse, coach, playground assistant) immediately when auto-injectable epinephrine is used
  - Not sharing medication with other students or leaving it unattended
  - Not using auto-injectable epinephrine for any other use than what is intended

For parents or guardians

- Desire for the student to self-carry and self-administer
- Awareness of school medication policies and parental responsibilities
- Commitment to making sure students have the needed medication with them, medications are refilled when needed, backup medications are provided, and medication use at school is monitored through collaborative effort between the parent or guardian and the school team

How does one know when a student is capable of self-treatment of an allergic reaction?

Most children over about age 7 can physically activate a self-injector, but no child should be depended on to do so in an emergency. If your school allows your child to self-carry, be sure to emphasize that this situation does not mitigate the need for an adult to take full responsibility for administering the medication in the event of an emergency. A survey of pediatric allergists suggested that they usually expect some transfer of responsibility by ages 12 to 14 years. However, there is no "correct" age for all children.

Some children may not be considered responsible enough to be carrying their medications because they tend to play with the medications and could injure themselves or another child. Other children may be responsible, but some of the children around them may not be and may take the medication if not supervised well enough, possibly risking injury. The answer also depends on a child's ability to understand the illness and appropriate treatment in the event of a reaction.

What is a 504 plan with regard to food allergy?

There is a public law (Section 504) that prohibits discrimination in education for any type of disability. The law applies to programs that receive federal funds and was developed for children with educational disabilities as well as vision and hearing impairment. The same law has been applied for children with other medical conditions, including allergies. Section 504 can be set up to require the school to have a plan that makes it safe for your child to attend the school and learn effectively as well as ensures that an emergency plan is in place; the plan can specify substitutions so that your child can participate in various activities with others.

Do I need a Section 504 plan to keep my child safe?

Most often, schools follow simple procedures and guidelines to ensure safety for children with food allergies without the need to invoke an individual Section 504 plan. Most of my patients do not develop 504 plans because they are able to obtain the needed accommodations for their child by discussing these needs with the administration and school nurse, providing a written emergency action plan that describes the allergy, and supplying the medications to treat a reaction. If you are having trouble with the school providing a safe environment, however, and the school receives federal funds, it is possible to set up a 504 plan to achieve the needed goals. The type of plan that is more directed to health issues, however, is the individualized health care plan.

What is an individualized health care plan (IHCP)?

The student's IHCP is typically developed by the school nurse in collaboration with the family, the child's physician, and other school personnel. The plan may include the emergency action plan that describes the allergy, symptoms, and treatments, as well as the means to avoid reactions, the roles of individuals in the child's care, and other aspects included in various state or national guidelines.

What special issues arise for college?

All the points made about school management, and food allergy management in general, apply in college except that the person with food allergies has more independent responsibility and will need to take more control of avoidance and treatment issues. Discuss food allergy management well ahead of college decision time. I recommend discussing college issues years in advance with your allergist. Many times, families and the student become interested in performing additional definitive diagnostic tests, such as the oral food challenge, prior to the student embarking on these last years toward independence. It is crucial to make sure the young adult knows how to avoid food allergens and how to self-treat in the event of anaphylaxis. Reading this book should help!

Are there colleges that specialize in students with food allergies?

Some colleges may have had more experience with students requiring special meals, but decisions about attending college should not be tied to food allergy, and most colleges are now capable of providing the necessary accommodations.

What living conditions at college should be addressed with regard to food allergy?

Meeting with food service personnel is important and might be arranged during preadmission visits. Personal preferences (living in a dormitory and having a meal plan versus living in housing with a kitchen and cooking for oneself) should be discussed. Roommates might be viewed as a liability if there is a shared kitchen because of cross-contact of allergens. However, having roommates has significant advantages for socialization and having others to watch out for the person with an allergy in the event of a reaction. Many schools have become significantly more allergy aware in the past several years, and programs are available to colleges regarding food allergen safety (for example, from www.foodallergy.org).

CAMP

What are some unique issues for staying safe with food allergies in camp?

All the same concerns for management in school apply to camps, as well as a few additional concerns:

- Supervising individuals may be young and inexperienced

- Activities may bring the child into remote areas (hikes)

- Attending overnight camps requires extensive provision of safe meals

Can a child with food allergies attend overnight camp?

Yes, as long as the concerns about allergen avoidance and recognition and treatment of an allergic reaction can be accommodated.

What are some hints to maintain safety in summer camps for children with food allergies?

- Discuss your child's food allergy well in advance, prior to committing to the experience.

- Ask what the camp has done in the past to manage children with food allergies.

- Discuss approaches that were successful at school and how they can be applied to the camp experience.

- Speak with food service personnel and camp health services.

- Review the camp's approaches to daily activities that affect food allergy management.

WORK

What are some unique concerns in the workplace for individuals with food allergy?

Co-workers may be less knowledgeable and understanding about food allergies. It may be difficult to maintain safe communal food areas. For example, a coffee maker might be used to make nut-flavored coffee, causing risks for an individual with nut allergies. Food storage or preparation areas might contain allergens. Thus, the allergic individual may need to take extra care in storing and preparing safe foods.

What type of food allergies are unique to the workplace?

Occupational food allergies most often develop in manufacturing plants or bakeries. Persons with baker's asthma can eat wheat but develop asthma symptoms when inhaling powdery flour during food preparation. Other airborne food proteins used in or caused by manufacturing include powdered milk and eggs, fish, and shellfish. Persistent itchy rashes from direct skin contact with food proteins can also occur.

What foods might cause skin reactions in the workplace?

For food handlers and manufacturers, the list of skin allergens and irritants is long. Some of the more common triggers are vegetables, fruits, raw fish, raw shellfish, raw meat, garlic, onion, seeds, and spices. Almost every food has caused some form of allergy for handlers in the workplace.

What are some tips to make the workplace safe for people with food allergies?
In food manufacturing settings, workers who are sensitive to the foods being worked with might wear goggles, masks, and gloves. Sometimes, occupational allergy to foods cannot be easily overcome and an alternative job must be sought.

For nonindustrial settings, an individual with food allergy must take care in food storage and preparation and be very cautious about ingesting foods from others who may not understand details about food allergen avoidance. For example, a well-meaning co-worker might make "nut-free" cookies but not understand the trace contamination introduced while preparing the food at home. Applying the "rules" about allergen avoidance described previously will promote safety in the workplace.

TRAVEL

What should I do to prepare for traveling safely with food allergies?
Avoiding an allergen during travel and vacation is similar to avoiding it in restaurants except there may be additional concerns, such as language barriers. Planning ahead is crucial to avoid mishaps. There are fewer options without the ability to prepare meals at home, so it may be helpful to consider lodging that offers a kitchenette. Call ahead to hotels and restaurants to discuss the allergy and ensure that there are safe options. Choose uncomplicated meals prepared simply to avoid cross-contact and hidden ingredients. Carry all medications and instructions. Be familiar with activating emergency services. Obtain location-specific allergy information (see chapter 11). Consider your destination's labeling laws (discussed earlier in this chapter).

How far from medical care can a person with food allergies be and still be safe?
Having a food allergy should not limit travel. Although it is ideal to be able to obtain advanced medical care quickly, for example, in less than 30 minutes, this may not be possible. If the travel is remote ensuring that all foods are entirely safe simply becomes more crucial.

How many epinephrine autoinjectors should I carry?

Typical instructions are to have two doses available at all times, so depending on the circumstances of the trip and considering that it may not be easy to refill a used autoinjector, it might be wise to carry at least one or two extra doses. More doses may be warranted for prolonged travel in remote areas.

Are there preferred, safe travel destinations for persons with food allergies?

Some destinations may be easier to manage. For example, a trip to a country where communication is limited would be much more difficult than one to a country where you can communicate fluently. Call ahead to theme parks because some are particularly allergy friendly. Disney has received awards from the Food Allergy & Anaphylaxis Network for its approach to food allergies, for example. With enough preparation, you should be able to travel without being excessively limited by food allergies.

What are the main concerns about airplane travel with food allergies?

Airplane travel can be anxiety provoking because of the isolation and distance from medical care. Persons with peanut allergies face the possibility of experiencing symptoms when many people in the cabin are opening powdery peanut snacks. The symptoms are usually mild. More severe symptoms are possible if the avoided food is eaten. Talk with your doctor about the potential risks as they apply to you or to your child's allergies and personal circumstances. Most of the time, the concerns would not warrant changing travel plans.

What are some strategies for traveling safely on airplanes with food allergy?

- Check the airline website for details about snacks, food for purchase, and what they serve. Also check the website www.foodallergy.org for updates on airline policies.

- Notify the airline about the allergy.

- Call ahead to the airline to discuss any special concerns.

- Obtain a note from your doctor indicating permission to carry medications and other supplies and foods because of the allergy (see chapter 11 for an example).

- Carry your medications and emergency action plan describing the allergy.
- Keep your medication in its original packaging, which includes prescription labels.
- Bring safe snacks and foods (do not trust the airline meals).
- Consider earlier flights when allergenic snacks may not be served.
- For young children with food allergies, check for leftover food on tray tables, in seat pockets, and in the seats, including cracks between seat cushions. Consider using a wet wipe on the seating and tray surfaces.

What are the primary concerns about travel on cruise ships with food allergies?
Similar to airplane travel, a cruise ship presents isolation from advanced medical care. Perhaps to a greater degree than other types of travel, there is dependence on others for providing safe foods. Therefore, it is recommended to call ahead to discuss your individual circumstances and ensure that safe meals will be obtainable.

DATING AND RELATIONSHIPS

Is it possible to have an allergic reaction from kissing?
Yes. About 10% of adults with food allergies describe having had such reactions, which are usually mild. They occur because residual protein in the saliva can be ingested through passionate kissing. An innocent kiss on the cheek is not likely to result in a significant reaction; more typically no symptoms are observed or at most, a localized swelling.

How can I reduce the risk of an allergic reaction from kissing?
We studied the time course of finding peanut protein in the saliva of people who ate an entire peanut butter sandwich. The amount of protein declined

rapidly in the hours after the sandwich. Brushing teeth, rinsing the mouth, and chewing gum all significantly reduced the amount of residual protein to levels not likely to cause severe reactions, but there was some residual protein. The most effective strategy was to allow about four hours to pass and to have had a peanut-free meal; in that situation we could not detect the peanut protein. This type of testing has not been tried with other foods, and presumably there is potential for solid bits of allergen, for example a tiny nut crumb, to dislodge from between teeth and cause a reaction in a partner. Therefore, the safest bet is to have an intimate partner avoid the allergen or at least eat a safe meal before passionate kissing.

Is it possible to have an allergic reaction from intercourse?

It is theoretically possible for food allergens to enter seminal fluid and potentially cause reactions in a sensitive partner. However, this has not been proven. There are rare case reports where allergic reactions to seminal fluids were attributed to foods or medications, but more often these reactions are due to actual allergy to the components of sperm and seminal fluids. Nonetheless, safety about kissing may apply to intercourse as well.

What are some tips to maintain safety for dating and relationships when there is food allergy?

It is particularly important to ensure that a partner is aware of the allergy so that precautions can be taken. Playing kissing games or indiscriminate intimacy with strangers or persons who are not aware of the allergy could have bad consequences for people with food allergies. Teenagers in particular should be aware of this concern.

AGE-RELATED RESPONSIBILITIES

How do food allergy management responsibilities change with age?

As children get older, they can take increasing responsibility for allergen avoidance and treatment of any reactions. The exact ages for transferring various responsibilities depend on personal factors, the family's comfort, and individual developmental factors. Talk to your child, doctor, teachers, and others to best understand what responsibilities should gradually be transferred.

How do I determine if my child can take on more responsibility for managing food allergies?

Observe your child in various situations to gauge readiness for increasing responsibility. Consider involving others, for example, to find out if your child will accept food from a stranger.

How do I encourage my child to become more independent with managing food allergies?

Reward successes and be positive about progress even if it appears that the transition is not imminent because of failures. The process should be consistent and gradual so that a teenager, based on years of experience, feels comfortable managing the allergies appropriately and experiences no awkwardness telling others about them.

What food allergy management responsibilities might be expected of a toddler?

Very few. This is a time to begin education. Introduce the concept of there being safe and unsafe foods. Try to use terms that are clear. For example, for a child with milk allergy, it is better practice to refer to "John's soy drink" rather than "John's special milk" to avoid misunderstandings about cow's milk versus soy "milk."

What food allergy management responsibilities might be expected of a preschool child?

At this age, the child should be taught that certain adults know what foods are safe. "Only Mom, Dad, Aunt Susie, and Grandma know what food you can eat safely. If you take food from other people, you could get sick." Although your child may know which foods to avoid, you should emphasize not accepting foods from people who are not "approved" by you. A preschooler may not be depended on to follow this rule and may grab foods, so constant supervision is needed.

**What food allergy management responsibilities might be expected of a
5- to 6-year-old?**

For this age group, continue to emphasize not taking foods unless approved by a responsible adult and expect your child to demonstrate this.
Some children begin to understand the role of emergency medications at
this age, but they are not usually ready to carry them responsibly. They
should be taught to report symptoms to an adult. This is a good age for
children to be taught how to comfortably inform others about their allergy.

**What food allergy management responsibilities might be expected of a
7- to 10-year-old?**

In this age group, children can partner with an adult to read ingredient
labels, choose safe foods, and talk about their allergies in restaurants. A
responsible adult still needs to oversee these actions and use this as a
learning time. Some children in this age group might be trusted to carry
medications but generally not to decide on when to use them.

**What food allergy management responsibilities might be expected of a
10- to 12-year-old?**

Under adult supervision, children in this age group should be capable of
discussing their allergies with restaurant personnel and correctly choos-
ing safe foods. If appropriate according to school regulations, they may
carry medications responsibly and should understand when to use them,
although they would not be depended on to do so.

**What food allergy management responsibilities might be expected of a
13- to 18-year-old?**

This is the age group when children are able to take responsibility for
obtaining safe meals and reporting and treating symptoms. However, this
is also an age of risk taking, so these responsibilities still require supervision. Teenagers should be frequently coached about their allergies and
treatment. These issues are discussed further in chapter 4.

SPECIAL EXPOSURE RISKS

As a breast-feeding mother, do I need to avoid eating foods my child is allergic to?

It depends, and this situation should be discussed with your child's allergist. The amount of allergen found in the breast milk is typically very low. It varies by individual and by how much was eaten. Allergy to foods in maternal breast milk has been linked to infants having flaring or eczema, mucous and blood stools (proctocolitis), and, very rarely, anaphylaxis.

What dietary options do I have while breast feeding my food-allergic child?

Options include strict avoidance, reduced ingestion, no change, or ingestion of specific forms of the food, for example, eggs or milk in bakery goods and not as whole milk or eggs. These considerations must be discussed with her doctor.

What factors might my allergist consider when deciding whether I should avoid eating the foods my child is allergic to while I'm still breast feeding?

We do not know if trace exposure to the allergen in breast milk speeds, hinders, or has no effect on a child's allergy recovery, so allergists primarily consider the risk of allergic reactions in the infant as well as nutritional and social factors for the mother.

If your child was perfectly fine on breast milk and had only mild symptoms when directly ingesting the food, you may not have to alter your diet or you may be advised not to exceed past amounts of ingestion. If your child had chronic symptoms when breast feeding, any sudden reactions to your breast milk after you ingested an allergen, or a severe reaction when ingesting the food directly, there is stronger reason for you to avoid the food in your own diet, or dramatically reduce ingestion.

The type of food involved is another consideration. For example, it may be easier and more prudent to avoid peanuts, nuts, fish, or shellfish for an infant diagnosed with these severe allergies, but if your child has a mild milk allergy, reducing your cow's milk consumption, or ingesting only baked forms, may be reasonable. Always talk to your allergist, and be sure to address nutritional issues if you need to avoid certain foods.

If I accidentally ate an allergen, such as peanuts, how long will it be in my breast milk?

This has not been extensively studied. In one small study, about half of mothers had detectable peanut in their breast milk after eating peanuts. It was usually found within two hours of ingestion and typically gone by eight hours, as tested by intermittent pumping.

Do medications contain food allergens?

They may, although this is not a common concern. Reports of allergic reactions to food proteins in medications are actually quite rare. The ingredients of medications are typically disclosed in package inserts, although not in the same manner as on food labels. Ask your pharmacist and allergist. In some cases, a call to the manufacturer is needed. Most medication flavoring is artificial, but it is sensible to check. Some types of inhaled asthma medications have been labeled as having soy lecithin. This is usually safe for persons with soy or peanut allergies, but ask your doctor to be sure. Coconut is a rare allergen, and coconut oil may have only trace proteins, but this is sometimes an ingredient in medications. Oils used in some medications are typically highly refined, and allergy risks are therefore minimal. Propofol, a type of injected anesthetic agent, has an ingredient derived from egg; there is no clear documented risk for persons with egg allergy, but if an alternative is easily obtained, this may avoid the theoretical risk. In all cases, discuss your particular concerns with your allergist.

Is lactose in medications a concern for those with milk allergy?

Pharmaceutical-grade lactose may sometimes contain trace residual milk proteins. You will need to ask your allergist if this is a concern. See chapter 1 for more information about this.

Do vaccines contain food allergens?

The measles, mumps, and rubella (MMR) vaccine is no longer considered a risk for persons with egg allergies. Seasonal influenza vaccines given by injection have a trace amount of egg that generally poses little risk. In most cases, your general physician will provide the vaccine and simply observe you for any problems for about 30 minutes. If you or your child has a severe egg allergy (more than just hives or stomach symptoms), your doctor may refer you to an allergist. The nasal vaccine has so far not been fully tested for safety in people with egg allergy. There may eventually be influenza vaccines without egg. The yellow fever vaccine, used for travelers to areas such as sub-Saharan Africa, has a greater amount of egg; if needed, an allergist can administer it in a graded fashion. Allergy to gelatin, derived from pork or beef bone, is rare but presents a risk for certain gelatin-containing vaccines. People with extremely severe milk allergies have been noted to react to booster doses of the diphtheria, pertussis, and tetanus combination vaccine (DPT), probably because some of the vaccine components are processed in materials derived from cow's milk. This appears to be rare but talk to your doctor.

Do hospitals understand how to prepare safe meals for someone with food allergies?

They should but do not assume so. Always check with the hospital personnel before eating meals (each one), and treat food services as you treat those serving you in a restaurant. See the section earlier in this chapter for ways to explain your allergy to those who prepare and serve your food.

Can blood transfusions trigger allergic reactions because of food allergy?

Theoretically, if a blood donor has eaten an allergen, it may appear in trace amounts in their bloodstream and be a problem for a recipient. When blood transfusions are processed, however, the liquid (serum) is washed away, so even if trace proteins had been in the blood donation, the amount left in the material that is transfused would be negligible. There have not been reports of reactions in this situation, although it may be reasonable for a donor providing a directed donation to a person with a food allergy to avoid the allergen for several hours prior to the donation. There is one report of a platelet donation causing a reaction in a child with peanut allergy (platelets are the blood-clotting component transfused without being separated from the serum). The report is not completely verified, but there may be a risk.

Delving Deeper:
RISKS AND RISK REDUCTION CONTROVERSIES

How worried should I be that my child will touch or smell an allergen and
develop an allergic reaction?

Anxiety and controversy surrounds the worry that smelling or touching
an allergen could result in a severe allergic reaction. Although there are
examples of foods becoming airborne during cooking or when they are
in a powdery form, the risks should be taken in context. A study that
purposefully aerosolized foods to which a child was allergic by cooking
them mostly found no reactions or only mild ones. Studies in which
peanut-allergic children smelled or were touched by peanut butter resulted in no reactions or in mild redness at the site of contact. There is
reason to have concern, but the anxiety about these exposures is probably
greater than the actual risks warrant. Talk to your doctor about the risks.
Your allergist might suggest a "test" of touching or smelling a food to
address your concerns.

Also of Interest:
THE PEANUT-SNIFFING DOG

What is a peanut-sniffing dog, and should I get one?

Trainers are selling dogs that can "sniff out" peanuts. Although there are
positive testimonials about this, my allergist colleagues and I have reser-
vations. First, the dogs are not able to accurately "approve" a safe meal,
which would perhaps be the most useful type of surveillance that is not
currently available (apart from asking questions about the food). Second,
because there are typically no significant risks of being *near* peanut as long
as the person is not eating peanut, the dog's main capability of identifying
nearby food is not crucial to avoiding eating the allergen. Third, relevant
allergen avoidance should emphasize label reading and asking questions
about foods in restaurants, not having a dog that cannot "test" the food it-

self, a situation that could result in a false sense of security. Fourth, having a dog only for peanut allergy avoidance presents a social and emotional factor that may seem empowering or comforting, but could also result in a feeling of vulnerability that is greater than necessary or result in isolation that is not necessary. Finally, allowing such a dog into schools or on planes may result in allergen exposure to persons with a dog dander allergy. If you are interested in this type of dog, talk to your allergist.

How Do I Manage a Food Allergy While Living a Normal and Healthy LIFESTYLE, with ADEQUATE NUTRITION?

This chapter answers questions about the daily lifestyle issues of living with food allergies. I explore emotional concerns and interpersonal relationships. I also explain nutritional management, including maintaining a healthy diet.

GENERAL QUESTIONS ON LIFESTYLE AND QUALITY OF LIFE

In what ways might food allergy affect lifestyle and health?

Living with food allergies can be limiting in many ways. Social occasions and each meal and snack present potential obstacles. Obtaining foods becomes time consuming. The burden on individuals and families can become great. Social activities and vacationing can be affected. Anxiety may increase because of the constant diligence and fear associated with each meal. Nutritional concerns may arise if the diet is limited, posing additional health concerns. Overall, social, emotional, and general health may be affected.

What is "health-related quality of life" as it relates to food allergy?

The term "health-related quality of life" refers to the impact that a health condition, in this case food allergy, may have on three major aspects of overall health: physical, social, and emotional or psychological well-being. Many people with food allergies "look fine," so it is often hard for people to understand the significant repercussions that living with a food allergy has on individuals and families. Studies I have performed show the effects as similar or even stronger than those of illnesses that the public recognizes as a burden, such as diabetes and severe arthritis.

Are there any simple ways to improve quality of life among people with food allergies?

A goal should be to ensure that the person with food allergies does everything that people without food allergies do except for eating the food to which they are allergic. Achieving this may not always be simple. The first step is to identify if there is a problem, and then to work with your health care professional to determine whether the trouble is

- related to concerns about food allergy or some other cause

- a reasonable or an excessive concern in relation to your allergies

- is treatable through simple education or requires more elaborate interventions

How might I know if food allergy is causing more of an impact on quality of life than it should?

Take time to discuss living with food allergies with your health care professional, even if you feel that you have everything under control. Sometimes you may be doing something you feel is warranted, that does not significantly affect your lifestyle, but that is actually unnecessarily limiting in comparison to how most people with food allergies live their lives.

For example, I was shocked to learn of a family who was having their child with food allergies eat in a room away from the rest of the family just because they thought this was a necessary routine. Other families might never go to a restaurant because of food allergies. These dramatic decisions are almost never necessary. The main point is to have a discussion with your doctor.

Consider the following questions. If your answer is "yes" to any of these, then address the concern with your doctor.

- Is there anything that the person with allergies would like to do but is not doing because of food allergies (aside from eating the avoided foods)?

- Does fear about food allergies result in altering the diet to avoid foods that should be safe to eat?

- Do emotional concerns about having a food allergy interfere with enjoying routine activities?

- Does fear of an allergic reaction result in altering daily routines in a way that is stressful or problematic?

- Is managing food allergies causing stresses that interfere with interpersonal relationships?

EMOTIONAL CONCERNS AND ANXIETY

What emotional concerns occur because of food allergies?
The most common emotion is anxiety. However, people with food allergies and their families may experience fear, sadness, depression, and many other negative emotions.

When should anxiety be considered a concern for people with food allergies?
The first step is to consider the degree of anxiety and its consequences. Food-allergic reactions are serious, so it is normal and healthy to have some anxiety. In fact, it may be protective by increasing vigilance. For example, if the anxiety motivates a person to check ingredient labels and ask appropriate questions in restaurants, that degree of anxiety is healthy.

Signs of unhealthy degrees of anxiety may come out in various ways:

- Concerns preventing you from eating in restaurants or at social functions

- Loss of sleep caused by thinking about your food allergy

- Rechecking foods you already checked and found safe

- Experiencing physical signs of anxiety and panic (sweating, shaking, heavy breathing, and so on) associated with meals and concerns about your food allergy

- Being in a heightened anxious state for more than a month after an allergic reaction

How should I address anxiety related to my food allergy?

Talk about the concern with your doctor. Anxiety disorders and phobias not related to food allergies can still affect food allergy management. It is helpful to diagnose this type of mental health problem because it can be treated and has no direct relationship to the food allergy. If the anxiety is solely related to your food allergy, learning more about it, with emphasis on what is and what is not worth worrying about may be helpful. For example, the unfounded worry that being near a food could cause a severe reaction may lead to unnecessary anxiety. Talk about your fears openly. When your anxiety is related to having experienced an allergic reaction, remember to focus on the positive aspects—that the reaction was recognized and treated, and that you learned from it. Sometimes additional tests, such as a food challenge or a "touch test" with a food, may allay concerns.

What is a "touch test" for food allergy?

I base the touch test on a study I performed with peanut butter. I had thirty children with severe peanut allergy sniff peanut butter for 10 minutes and I touched them with a pea-sized amount of peanut butter for a minute. None of the children had a reaction to smelling the peanut butter (one had an anxiety response when smelling fake peanut butter used as a placebo) and none had more than a minor itch or redness at the spot the peanut butter touched. Afterward, many of the children and families felt less worried about being around the food. I have since used these touch tests to help reduce fears about casual exposures. Talk to your allergist about this.

Can anxiety cause food allergy?

Anxiety itself does not cause the body to have a food allergy, but it can result in symptoms that mimic a food allergy. One way this can occur is through hyperventilation.

How does hyperventilation mimic a food allergy reaction?

When people become fearful and anxious, they may not notice that they are breathing deeply and rapidly. Doing so alters the chemicals in the bloodstream, which can result in light-headedness, muscle cramps, tingling, numb fingers, and feeling as though they are having trouble breathing. It can be difficult to know whether the symptoms are from hyperventilation or an allergic reaction when fear of a food exposure is part of the reason for the anxiety. I think that explaining this situation to people who have been having such symptoms often improves the problem through awareness. Anxiety counseling may be needed as well.

Is there a link between food allergy and mental health problems?

There is no clear link between mental health disorders and food allergies. Some controversial reports link food allergies with depression, but more studies are needed.

Can food-allergic reactions cause increased anxiety?

Yes. An allergic reaction can be a scary event that might cause increased anxiety for a time. This anxiety should naturally wane in days or weeks. If it does not, talk to your doctor. Sometimes a traumatic life event will lead to a more severe form of anxiety, a post-traumatic stress disorder.

Can food-allergic reactions result in fear of eating?

Yes. Sometimes people with food allergies begin to distrust the safety of various foods and may excessively limit their diet. Although this is a protective response, it is an example of an over-reaction. Talk to your doctor about this if it should occur. Counseling is beneficial.

How should I address resistance to eating caused by anxiety in a child with a food allergy?

For a child, it should be helpful to emphasize that the responsible adults are checking to make sure the foods are as safe as possible. Depending on the degree of concern and resistance in eating, it may be necessary to gradually reexpand the diet over weeks. Provide positive reinforcement. For a child, this may be a sticker chart, with a sticker for each small gain and rewards every so often for progress. Rewards should be given for even the smallest successes, and no one should dwell on times when progress is not made.

How should I address resistance to eating caused by anxiety in an adult with a food allergy?

For an adult, excessive dietary restriction may require a multidisciplinary approach, with counselors, allergists, and trusted friends ensuring that the diet is appropriately and safely expanded.

How can I handle sadness and depression related to food allergy?

It is normal to feel sad, helpless, or angry because of food allergies. It is not "fair" to have dietary restrictions and the constant concerns about allergic reactions. Also normal are feelings of guilt that arise among family members, who may feel as though they somehow caused the allergy. Some feel lucky not to have a food allergy, and then feel guilty for even thinking that. All of these feelings, if periodic and not interruptive of daily activity and social interactions, are normal. Talk about these feelings with friends, relatives, clergy, and professionals as needed. If the feelings are constant, overwhelming, or interruptive, however, you should seek professional assistance.

How should I address my general well-being as it relates to food allergy?

Although it is normal and expected that having food allergies, or having a family member with them, will result in concerns about general well-being, these feelings should not interfere with daily activities. Remember that people with food allergies can live full and happy lives while taking the necessary precautions to stay safe. This is the aspect that should be emphasized.

Is there a way to prevent anxiety, fear, and depression related to food allergies?

Not entirely, but there are healthy approaches that should reduce the risk of an over-reactive response to having a food allergy.

- Focus on the individual's positive traits. A person is not to be defined by their having a food allergy. They are smart, creative, warm, friendly, artistic, athletic, compassionate, altruistic, and so on.

- Focus on allergy management successes. Emphasize the successfully obtained restaurant meal, the persistence in ensuring that activities are not curtailed by having food allergies.

- Address concerns early. If anxieties and fears are resulting in unnecessary alterations in lifestyle, address the problem quickly before poor habits set in.

- Avoid anxiety-provoking discussions around young children. Do not discuss dying from food allergies, turning blue, the throat closing, or other scary terms. It is less troubling to use terms such as "could make you sick."

- Talk to your doctor about what you should and should not be concerned about. It is anxiety provoking to be fearful of trace exposures that cannot be seen. Do you or your child need to be concerned about ingesting trace amounts? Do you or your child need to be concerned about touching or being near the allergens? Usually the answer to these questions is "no," and this could allay anxiety.

When is it time to get professional mental health services to address problems caused by dealing with a food allergy?

In our studies, over 75% of people living with food allergies said they would benefit from mental health counseling. This high number reflects how difficult managing food allergies can be. Numerous studies have shown a significant change in quality of life. If you or your family are experiencing frequent and disruptive emotional concerns, discuss this with your doctor and consider professional mental health services.

How would I recognize emotional concerns or anxiety in a very young child?

A young child might have changes in behavior after an allergic reaction or another life event. The changes could be alterations in sleep patterns, increased aggression, defiance, expressions of sadness, reduced activities with family and friends, expression of worries, and changes in eating. Discussion with your physician and referral to a mental health professional are options. Various techniques for counseling and therapy are available, including play therapy (www.a4pt.org).

Can food allergy cause mental illnesses like depression or schizophrenia?
No. There are some who hold the belief that foods cause various mental health problems through "allergy" or other effects. There are no proven direct links. You should discuss these concerns with a physician or mental health professional, because altering the diet rather than addressing the problem through proper treatment can result in delaying effective treatment.

INTERPERSONAL RELATIONSHIPS AND BULLYING

How do I address family relationships affected by food allergies?
It is not uncommon for management of food allergies to result in frustration among family members. Siblings may feel limitations caused by the diet restrictions. Relatives might not show the support that was hoped for in providing a safe environment. Sometimes relatives respond with disbelief about the allergy or feel that it should be addressed with less or more restrictions. Making sure everyone involved is fully educated about the allergy is helpful, especially to address questions about managing the allergy. The activities of siblings and other family members do not usually need to be restricted, but if this becomes necessary, it is fair to provide special occasions for them so that all the attention is not constantly focused on the allergy.

How should I address spousal relations that are affected by our child's food allergy?
Marital stress associated with managing a child's food allergies is common. Different parenting styles, varying levels of concern, or divergent preferences for managing the allergy can all put a strain on the relation-

ship. If at all possible, both parents should attend office visits with the allergist to ask questions and determine approaches to care that are agreeable and safe. Talk about the disagreements without involving your child, then favor a unified approach once the disagreements are aired.

How common is bullying of children with food allergies compared with those who don't have them?
Our study showed that 50% of children with food allergies in grades 6 through 10 had experienced bullying, teasing, or harassment, compared with 17% without food allergies. The bullying was generally along the lines of taunting ("Ha, ha, I'm eating this, and you can't have any!"), provoking fear ("You drank from the water fountain after I rubbed peanut butter on it!"), or physical abuse (e.g., throwing peanuts, tainting a meal with allergen). Bullying has most often been attributed to peers, but adults and others may also be the perpetrators.

What are the negative consequences of bullying for a child with food allergies?
Being bullied does not make a person "stronger." Depression, low self-esteem, health issues, poor grades, and suicidal ideations are potential results of this victimization. For children with food allergies, the impact of bullying may be increased by the risks of a reaction when physical threats are involved.

Why is bullying more common for children with food allergies?
One possibility is that other children, or adults, are curious about the allergy and test boundaries.

How should bullying of children with food allergies be addressed?
Studies show that a child may not inform parents about food-related bullying, so parents need to raise the issue and discuss it with their child.

Many schools have general programs to address bullying or will invoke state laws on the subject. The following advice is based on articles written by Mati Sicherer, M.A., a school counselor with expertise in bullying:

1. Recognize signs of bullying, including torn clothing or damaged books; unexplained injuries; school avoidance; physical complaints

(headaches or stomachaches; consistent nightmares; lower grades and loss of interest in schoolwork; change in demeanor, with sadness or outbursts; and social isolation).

2. Be responsive and listen to your child. Stay calm. Reassure your child that you will help with this problem.

3. Do not confront the bully yourself. Parental intervention in bullying situations tends to exacerbate the problem. The school personnel are the appropriate ones to have primary responsibility for managing the bully.

4. Do not encourage retaliation. Teaching your child to tease or fight back typically makes the situation worse. The bully is unlikely to be stopped by your child's response. Bullying is based on an inequity of power, so recurrent conflict allows the bully to display strength over your child. Encourage reduced contact with the bully.

5. Teach your child the difference between "telling" and "tattling." "Tattling" is done to get someone in trouble, while "telling" is done to get help. Encourage your child to promptly "tell" an adult about bullying.

6. Although the weight of responsibility should not be placed on your child, be proactive and teach assertive social skills. Role-play and practice ways to deal with the bully. Teaching your child how to say "Leave me alone" in a confident manner may be all it takes to stop a bully.

7. Inform and involve teachers, the principal, and other school staff. Do not assume that they know about the bullying. Many times, victims do not want to tell for fear of retaliation.

8. Set up a buddy system. Encourage your child to stay in a group of trusted friends in high-risk areas, such as the lunchroom, during recess, and on the walk home from school.

9. Encourage educational programs about food allergy and about bullying. Teachers, counselors, and the school nurse may be able to provide lessons to increase food allergy awareness and reduce bullying.

10. Talk to your child's principal or school counselor about policies and plans regarding bullying. A typical approach is to initially observe the situation for a brief time and then take action. Serious consequences for the bully should be a part of the plan. Simple things such as moving the bully away from your child in class, not placing the bully in your child's class the following year, and staggering leaving times for the two children can be effective.

NUTRITION

What nutritional concerns arise for an individual living with food allergies?
Depending on the number of foods avoided, concerns include whether there are sufficient calories, protein, carbohydrates, vitamins, minerals, and micronutrients (trace elements) in the diet.

Do food allergies cause weight gain or obesity?
No. There is a notion in the popular press that allergy, such as allergy to wheat, causes weight gain. Although avoiding wheat products such as cakes, cookies, and pasta might result in weight loss, this is not a sign of a true allergy.

Can food allergies cause weight loss or poor weight gain?
Yes, with three possible explanations: if there is inadequate energy (calorie) intake, increased energy needs that are not being met, or poor absorption of ingested calories.

Why would food allergies cause inadequate calorie intake?
Several reasons. There could be inadequate replacement of alternative foods during avoidance diets. Some illnesses may result in poor appetite and lower intake (for example, eosinophilic esophagitis). Sometimes anxiety about eating results in food avoidance or refusal or very limited dietary intake.

Why would food allergies cause increased energy needs?
If there are severe skin rashes or inflammation of the gut, the body may need extra calories to make constant repairs.

Why would food allergy result in poor absorption of calories?
If allergens are causing inflammation in the gut, there can be reduced efficiency of the gut in absorbing needed nutrients.

Can food allergies cause poor growth in children?
Yes. Usually there is poor weight gain ahead of any reduction in height. There should be room for "catch-up" when the problem is recognized and addressed.

Are nutritional requirements different for people with food allergies?
No, but if there is ongoing severe eczema (atopic dermatitis), the child may require extra calories to continuously repair the skin damage. If gut allergies are causing poor nutrient absorption, additional nutrients may be needed until the digestive system heals.

What type of nutritional monitoring is recommended for persons on a food allergy elimination diet?
For children, their height and weight should be monitored on standard growth curves.

What nutrients are needed in the diet?
A healthy diet includes a proper amount of protein, fat, carbohydrates, vitamins, minerals, and trace elements. Caloric intake, the amount of energy from the diet, is an important consideration for proper growth. Calories are derived from the intake of protein, fat, and carbohydrates. In addition to energy, specific nutrients (vitamins, minerals) in the diet are needed to ensure proper body functions and to prevent illness.

Why are proteins needed, and how does food allergy affect protein intake?
Proteins are a source of the building blocks of life, amino acids. Good quality proteins that include specific, much-needed "essential" amino acids

are typically obtained from meats or complementary foods, the classic rice and beans, for individuals who are vegetarian or allergic.

What fats are needed in the diet and how does food allergy affect fat intake?

Fats are a major source of calories, and essential fatty acids (linoleic and linolenic) are necessary for proper brain development in infants. These types of essential fatty acids are found in fish, which is often excluded from the diet of an individual with food allergy. These fatty acids are also available in vegetable oils, such as canola, corn, soy, safflower, and olive. The diet should consists of a blend of saturated fats, which are usually of animal origin, and monounsaturated and polyunsaturated fats, which are components of vegetable oils.

What carbohydrates are needed in the diet, and how might food allergy affect carbohydrate intake?

Carbohydrates, or complex sugars, are a major source of calories needed for growth, generally accounting for nearly half of the caloric intake. Vegetables, fruits, and grains contain carbohydrates. Wheat products are a common source of carbohydrates, but this food is a common food allergy. Substitutions for carbohydrates could, therefore, include rice, oats, potatoes, corn, and quinoa.

What additional dietary nutrients are needed in the diet?

Vitamins, minerals, and trace elements are necessary for various functions in the body, such as blood clotting, bone development, teeth development, proper nerve and muscle function, and many others. Examples of vitamins are vitamin A, which helps with growth and night vision, and vitamin D, which aids in the body's use of calcium. Examples of minerals are calcium, for bone development, and iron, for the blood. Trace elements in the body include zinc, which is needed for healing and immune function.

What is the role of vitamin D in allergy?

Studies suggest that vitamin D deficiency may be a risk factor for allergy and that people with allergies may be more likely to be deficient. There is some evidence that vitamin D is needed to promote healthy immune responses. This does not mean that taking excessive supplemental vitamin D is warranted. Doing this could in fact be detrimental. The body naturally makes vitamin D when exposed to sunlight, and vitamin D is in many foods, but some of them are common allergens (milk, fish, eggs). Talk to your doctor about whether a blood test to check your or your child's vitamin D level is warranted.

What are alternative sources of nutrition for people avoiding allergens?

If you or your child are avoiding several foods, you should discuss your specific dietary needs with your doctor and possibly a registered dietitian. For younger children, complete formulas are available to supplement any potential deficiency. The table on page 211 provides some examples of nutrients that may be affected by allergen elimination and suggests alternatives.

Keep in mind that the amount of nutrients in the alternative sources may vary greatly. For example, a calcium-fortified soy drink may or may not have "ounce for ounce" calcium levels similar to milk, and a calcium-fortified beverage likely has much more calcium per serving than a vegetable does. Be sure to discuss these substitutions with your doctor or dietitian.

How much carbohydrate, protein, fat, and other nutrients do I need for a healthy diet?

This varies with age. The United States Department of Agriculture (USDA) maintains consumer-friendly documents regarding dietary recommendations at www.usda.gov. You can also check www.choosemyplate.gov.

Will my child get enough calcium on a milk-restricted diet?

Many beverages are calcium fortified. Usually children are not allergic to the various calcium-fortified fruit juices available, but calcium-fortified soy or rice drinks would also be a good choice and often have more calcium than the juices. It may be necessary to provide calcium as a supplement, for example, calcium carbonate tablets. Calcium and vitamin D needs change with age, so talk to your doctor or dietitian.

Table 7.1
Nutrients affected by allergen elimination—and alternative sources of those nutrients

Nutrient	Allergen	Alternative sources
Vitamin A	Milk	Spinach, potatoes, squash, carrots
Vitamin D	Milk	Fortified alternative "milks" and juices, margarine
Vitamin E	Peanut	Green leafy vegetables, vegetable oils, grains
Thiamin	Soy, wheat	Pork, beef, beans, grains
Riboflavin	Milk, egg, soy, wheat	Meats, leafy green vegetables, grains
Niacin	Wheat, peanut	Meats, beans, enriched grains
Vitamin B12	Milk, egg	Meats
Folate	Soy	Leafy green vegetables, beans
Pantothenic acid	Milk, egg	Meats, fruits, vegetables, grains
Calcium	Milk	Leafy green vegetables, beans, calcium-fortified drinks
Chromium	Peanut	Whole grains
Iron	Wheat, soy	Meats, beans, dried fruits, iron-fortified grains
Magnesium	Soy, peanut	Fruits, vegetables, grains
Manganese	Peanut	Leafy green vegetables, whole grains
Phosphorus	Milk, soy	Poultry meats, carbonated beverages
Selenium	Egg	Meats, grains
Zinc	Soy	Meats, beans

Does using soy drinks cause problems in boys?

There is some concern that phytoestrogens (plant-derived estrogens) as found in soy may have negative effects on men or boys. At this time, research studies fail to support this worry, and various professional organizations and government agencies have concluded that there is no concern.

Does food allergy cause picky eating in children?

No. Many young children have narrow food preferences with or without food allergies.

When should consultation with a registered dietitian be undertaken for food allergy?

If there is any concern about a growth deficiency or when prolonged dietary avoidance is undertaken, a consultation makes good sense. Since nutrient deficiency could occur despite normal growth, consider contacting a dietitian if the diet is devoid of several common foods or if there is any suspicion that a restricted diet may be nutritionally inadequate.

What are the benefits of a nutritional evaluation for persons with food allergy?

There are several. The dietitian may have advice about products that are free from your or your child's allergens. The dietitian can also review a three- to seven-day diet record to determine if you or your child is obtaining the appropriate calories and balance of protein, carbohydrates, fats, vitamins, minerals, and trace elements needed for proper growth, health, and development. If there are potential deficiencies, substitutions could be suggested, such as using additional oils or seeking supplements in the form of multivitamins, iron, or calcium. Of course, it is vital to review with your dietitian the specific food allergies, so the substitute foods are appropriately selected.

Delving Deeper:
AN ALLERGIC REACTION'S EFFECT ON QUALITY OF LIFE

Could having an allergic reaction improve quality of life?

Yes. You would think that a food-allergic reaction would mostly increase anxiety, and it could, but some studies looking at doctor-supervised feeding tests (oral food challenges) showed improvement in measurements of quality of life whether or not the test resulted in a reaction. This could be because the person experiencing the reaction learned that (1) they are avoiding the food for a good reason, and (2) the reaction symptoms were recognizable and manageable, countering anxiety about what a food-allergic reaction might entail.

Also of Interest:
ANXIETY REACTIONS

Can anxiety cause a person to appear to have a food-allergic reaction?

Absolutely. This is a reason why doctor-supervised feeding tests are sometimes designed to include placebo food, which does not contain the allergen being tested but looks, tastes, and smells like the real thing. This allows the testing to proceed with less bias. It can be very difficult for a doctor or a person with a food allergy to know if symptoms are from anxiety or a true reaction. Anxiety symptoms can include changes in skin color, trouble breathing, throat tightness, sweating, vomiting, and loss of consciousness. These symptoms clearly overlap those of an allergic reaction.

The reason for anxiety is clear. Your body knows to fear the food that can cause a reaction. If I held a loaded gun to your head, you might shake, sweat, turn pale, have trouble catching your breath, and even pass out—clearly not from a gun allergy but out of fear and anxiety. This is a normal protective neurologic and hormonal reaction, but it can complicate food allergy diagnosis and treatment. If you or your doctor suspect anxiety reactions, this problem should be openly discussed and evaluated, and referral to a mental health professional should be considered.

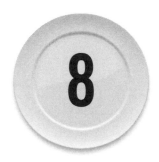

8

Will These Food Allergies
Ever GO AWAY?

This chapter answers your questions about whether your food allergy is likely to resolve and how the natural course of an allergy varies for different foods.

GENERAL QUESTIONS ABOUT FOOD ALLERGY RESOLUTION

Can food allergies resolve?
Yes.

Which food allergies are most likely to resolve?
Childhood allergies to milk, egg, wheat, and soy typically resolve.

Which food allergies are typically long-lived?
Allergies to peanuts, tree nuts, fish, and shellfish are typically persistent.

Why is a food allergy outgrown?
We do not know. Some theories are discussed in the "Delving Deeper" section near the end of this chapter.

What predicts whether a food allergy will resolve?

There are no simple predictors, although having relatively lower food-specific IgE-antibody levels in the blood is associated with a better chance of the allergy resolving.

Is there anything that can speed recovery from a food allergy?

The answer to this question is elusive. Some believe that strict avoidance speeds recovery, but this idea remains unproven. Children with milk or egg allergy who can tolerate small amounts of these foods when they are extensively heated in baked goods, such as muffins, appear to have an increased chance to outgrow milk and egg allergies. Some children have anaphylaxis to these types of baked foods, so talk to your doctor.

THE COURSE OF ALLERGIES TO SPECIFIC FOODS

What is the natural course of peanut allergy?

This allergy is usually long-lived, although about 20% of children under age 2 with a peanut allergy will outgrow it by adolescence.

What is the natural course of tree nut allergies?

Allergies to tree nuts are usually long-lived, but 5% to 10% of children diagnosed under age 2 will outgrow it by adolescence.

What is the natural course of milk allergy?

Milk allergy usually resolves in childhood. There is a very good chance (about 80%) that the allergy will resolve before age 5, although some recent studies suggest that the rate of outgrowing milk allergy has slowed, with about half still allergic around age 8. Nonetheless, most children outgrow this allergy by adolescence.

What is the natural course of egg allergy?

Egg allergy usually resolves in childhood. There is a very good chance (about 80%) that the allergy will resolve before age 5, although some recent studies suggest that the rate of outgrowing egg allergy has slowed, with about half still allergic around age 10. Nonetheless, most children outgrow this allergy by adolescence.

What is the natural course of soy allergy?

Soy allergy usually resolves in childhood. There is a very good chance (about 85%) that the allergy will resolve before age 5, although some recent studies suggest that the rate of outgrowing soy allergy has slowed, with about half still allergic around age 7. Nonetheless, most children outgrow this allergy by adolescence.

What is the natural course of wheat allergy?

Wheat allergy usually resolves in childhood. There is a very good chance (about 85%) that the allergy will resolve before age 5, although some recent studies suggest that the rate of outgrowing wheat allergy has slowed, with about half still allergic around age 6. Nonetheless, most children outgrow this allergy by adolescence.

What is the natural course of fruit and vegetable allergy?

Most fruit and vegetable allergies are associated with pollen allergies. They are usually mild, occur with the raw forms, and occur throughout adulthood. They can vary significantly depending on the pollen season, with more abundant pollen seasons triggering more symptoms when the fruit or vegetable is eaten. The natural course has not been studied well but likely varies significantly depending on pollen exposure.

What is the natural course of meat allergy?

This has not been studied, but it is possible to outgrow a meat allergy.

What is the natural course of fish and shellfish allergies?

These allergies are usually long-lived. The rate of resolution has not been studied well but is probably in the range of 5% to 10%.

THE COURSE OF ILLNESSES CAUSED BY FOOD ALLERGIES

Do food allergies that cause food protein–enterocolitis syndrome (FPIES) resolve?

Most often these resolve within a few years. Unfortunately, a small percentage of people continue to have this type of allergy for many, many years.

Do food allergies causing eosinophilic esophagitis resolve?

Eosinophilic esophagitis appears to be a chronic disease that is usually not completely outgrown. The triggering foods could vary over time, so periodic reassessment is necessary.

Do food allergies causing anaphylaxis resolve?

Yes, they can, according to the course of allergy associated with the individual food.

Does food-associated exercise-induced anaphylaxis resolve?

There are no good studies on this question. It may be related to the course of allergy to the causal food.

Does oral allergy syndrome resolve?

It varies in severity and triggers over time, but no studies detail how often the problem resolves completely.

Does atopic dermatitis (eczema) related to foods resolve?

Based on observations that food triggers of atopic dermatitis are uncommon among adults, it seems that this problem often resolves during childhood.

EVALUATIONS FOR RESOLUTION OF FOOD ALLERGY

How does one know when a food allergy is outgrown?
The allergist performs tests to monitor for improvement. At some point, if there is significant improvement, a medically supervised feeding test could be performed to determine resolution. This test may also be offered if a circumstance indicates that the allergy might have resolved; for example if an accidental ingestion did not result in any reaction.

What tests are performed to monitor for resolution of food allergy?
The two main tests are skin tests and blood tests measuring the food-specific IgE antibodies. To monitor an allergy, the blood test is most convenient. Decreasing test results are often a good sign that the allergy is resolving, although for young children, having results not increase is also a good sign. See chapter 3 for more details about allergy testing.

Why would a food allergy test increase or decrease?
We often see this despite no clear explanation. This question is addressed in detail in chapter 3.

How often should allergy testing be done to evaluate for resolution?
The factors that an allergist considers in retesting include the age of the child, the food involved, the time since the last reaction, and personal preferences and curiosity. Younger children might be tested with a higher frequency (perhaps every 6 to 12 months) than older persons because changes occur more rapidly. Some foods that are outgrown more readily, such as milk, eggs, wheat, and soy, might be tested more often than foods that tend to cause persistent allergies, such as peanuts, nuts, fish, and shellfish.

RECURRENCE OF A FOOD ALLERGY AND DEVELOPMENT OF NEW FOOD ALLERGIES

Is it possible to redevelop a food allergy that is outgrown?
Yes, but this is unusual. A medically supervised feeding test is typically performed to confirm that a food allergy has resolved. Once a person has "passed" a medically supervised feeding of a food, they are generally able to eat that food for life. About 2% of the time, the test appears to have resulted in no symptoms but problems arise in the days following. That is different from a situation in which a person who passed the feeding test has successfully consumed the food many times since. Once an individual is routinely eating the food, it is very unusual to have the food allergy recur.

Under what circumstances have food allergies redeveloped after resolution?
Since it is possible to develop a new food allergy at any time of life, an allergy that was outgrown could recur, although this is rare. One food to which recurrence of allergy has been well documented are peanuts. Almost all recurrences of peanut allergy happened under similar circumstances. The individual successfully ingested peanuts during a feeding test but did not continue to incorporate peanuts in their diet afterward. They noticed symptoms many months or over a year later when they tried to eat peanuts again.

If a food allergy resolved, how often does the food need to be eaten to prevent recurrence?
Although our experience with peanuts suggests that continuing to eat the food may be important, there are no established guidelines. I do not suggest creating a calendar for eating a food. Rather, when a new food is added to the diet after an allergy has resolved, incorporate it into the diet in a way that it would be naturally. For peanuts this might be a few times a month, and for foods like milk and eggs, it would be many times each week.

Why does a new food allergy occur in adults?

We do not know, but there are theories. The most common new allergy is to proteins in airborne allergens such as pollens. These proteins are similar to those in various fruits and vegetables. Exposure to an airborne protein seems to trigger an allergy more often than exposure to an ingested protein, which may explain this situation. One theory suggests that the adult's immune system might become vulnerable for a period after a viral infection or other illness. Still other theories suggest that changes in digestion may create a vulnerability. No one knows for certain why new allergies develop.

Which food allergies are more common to develop in adulthood?

Allergies to fruits and vegetables. Next most common are allergies to seafood and to tree nuts.

FACTORS AFFECTING THE COURSE OF FOOD ALLERGIES

Does the severity of an allergy affect resolution?

The answer to this is somewhat unclear because many children with severe reactions to foods such as egg, milk, wheat, and soy nonetheless outgrow these allergies. Compared with children who have consistently milder symptoms, however, persons experiencing more severe reactions, especially if they have strong positive tests, seem to experience a longer lived allergy.

Does being exposed to an allergen or having reactions affect the natural course?

Although it might be assumed that having exposures prolongs the allergy, this is not proved. On the one hand, some studies show that recurrent exposures heighten allergic responses. On the other hand, studies aimed to treat food allergy have used exposure to attempt to reduce the allergic response. In a practical sense, a person with allergies must take all necessary precautions to avoid exposure, but I would not consider an accidental ingestion or purposeful exposure during food challenges to significantly change the possibility of outgrowing allergy.

Delving Deeper:
RESOLUTION OF FOOD ALLERGIES

Why do allergies resolve?

The immune system is supposed to recognize, but generally ignore, the proteins in our foods. When a food allergy resolves, perhaps the immune system has altered the way it was recognizing the food. This might be because the immune system's cells eventually forget about attacking the protein. For example, vaccines given to fight infection alert an immune response against the germ. After some time, for many types of vaccines, this protection goes away and the person needs to be revaccinated to alert the immune system to remember to attack the germ. Perhaps after time away from the allergenic food, the misdirected attack on it is forgotten.

Another possibility is that the immune system has some chances to see the food protein again but does so in a healthier way. Perhaps during a time of earlier exposure, the immune system was irritable and set to attack the new food and later is behaving appropriately and learns to ignore the food. Yet another possibility has to do with the way the food is digested. An infant's gut may be more prone to let food proteins pass into the bloodstream. If the immune system is attacking undigested proteins, but ignores digested ones, which often may be the case, then a child may outgrow their food allergy primarily because they are digesting the foods more effectively.

Also of Interest:
THE AIR-FOOD CONNECTION

How can noningestion exposure to foods cause new food allergies?
The explanation for infant and child food allergy usually includes an immaturity of the immune system and gut. For adults, whose immune systems are supposed to be able to recognize but intelligently ignore food proteins, there often appears to be a possibility of becoming allergic because of airborne exposure. An example is baker's asthma, where occupational exposure to wheat protein results in wheat-induced asthma.

Another example is oral allergy syndrome, or pollen-associated allergy syndrome, where allergy to pollen results in symptoms from raw fruits or vegetables that have similar proteins inside them. Curiously, other environmental allergens share similar proteins to foods. Many tree nuts also have pollen-related proteins. Shellfish share proteins with dust mites and cockroaches, which are common environmental allergens. No one knows for certain, but this may be one reason that adults are more likely to develop these allergies, especially to foods that are eaten infrequently. The immune system may have time to develop an attack from the respiratory side while the gut side of the immune system is not being exposed. In the next chapter I discuss how skin exposure to foods may be related to developing food allergies.

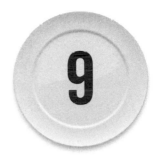

Is There Any Way to
PREVENT Food Allergies?

In this chapter, I address questions about risk factors for food allergy and how we may be able to prevent food and other allergic illnesses by reducing those risks.

GENERAL QUESTIONS ON PREVENTION

Is there anything good about having allergies that would deter us from preventing them?

A stuffy nose in the pollen season might help to filter a little more pollen, and an asthma cough might help to blow out extra debris from our lungs, but it is hard to imagine these symptoms are particularly good for us, and certainly food allergies can be deadly. It would therefore be great if we could prevent these problems.

Why would the body do something that can hurt us, like attack foods?

The immune system, the part of the body that typically fights infection, is responsible for causing allergies, including those to food. The cells and chemicals that are designed to combat parasite or worm infections are also the ones that trigger allergies. Therefore, a food allergy can be thought of as a misdirected response against foods from a part of the body that is ready to fight germs, especially parasites.

Why would the immune system turn against us by attacking foods?

The "hygiene hypothesis" is one theory for this, that our clean lifestyle has left our immune systems without much need to fight infections, making them more likely to attack innocent proteins, resulting in allergy. We have avoided germs by living in cities rather than on farms, having smaller families and larger living spaces that reduce exposure to germs, living in clean houses and apartments, and using vaccinations, antibiotics, soaps, and other measures to stay healthy. Birth by Caesarean section may increase risk of developing allergies because the infant does not have exposure to the natural bacteria of the birth canal. Most of all, we have protected ourselves from parasite infections. Persons who are prone to allergy may have immune systems that would be very effective fighting against parasites.

Can we learn how to prevent food allergies from the people who do not get them?

Yes! But first we have to consider *why* people develop food allergies. Genetics and environment are both responsible.

How does genetics influence having a food allergy?

Genetics, or heredity, is how we pass along traits such as hair or eye color. Heredity is also important for allergy. It cannot be changed, but knowing the genetic risk of allergy can help focus prevention toward people who are at greater risk. Allergies are more likely to occur in a person whose relatives have allergic diseases, such as asthma, eczema, hay fever, or food allergies. The more types of allergies, and the more relatives with allergies, the more likely another family member will have them.

What is the risk of allergy in a child born in a family with allergies?

Considering any allergic problem, there is roughly a 15% risk to a child if there is just a sibling with allergies, a 30% risk if one parent, and a 50% risk if both parents have allergies. Specific allergic diseases run in families as well. There is over a 50% risk of asthma for a child if both parents have asthma.

What is the risk of "inheriting" food allergies?

We do not know the exact risk of inheriting allergies to specific foods. My studies found that siblings have a 7% risk of sharing a peanut allergy, which is about seven times higher than expected. Still, a person with allergies often has no relatives who are also suffering.

If a person has nonfood allergies, are they at more risk of having a food allergy as well?

A personal history of any allergy increases an individual's risk for having additional allergies. The more allergic diseases, or the more severe the allergic disease, the more likely a food allergy will occur. My studies found that if a child's allergic eczema is moderate or severe—if half the body or more is affected with the persistent rash—there is about a 35% risk of developing a food allergy.

What role does dietary exposure play in the risk of having a food allergy?

Although genetics is key, environment clearly plays a role. More exposure to a food allergen is a large part of the risk of having an allergy. You probably do not know anyone who is allergic to sluremi. The reason is that there is no such food as sluremi, and therefore no one can have an allergy to it. Acorn nuts would probably be a significant allergen, but they are too sour to eat and so allergy is not an issue (except, perhaps, for squirrels!). Allergy to rice is much more common in Japan than in the United States, which probably reflects Japan's higher rice consumption. Kiwi allergy was not described in the United States until these fruits were imported.

How strong a role does the environment or diet play in the risk of having a food allergy?

A very strong role. In my study of identical twins who share the same genes, only two-thirds shared peanut allergy. If genes were the whole story, the rate of shared allergy would be 100%. Some type of environmental exposure was responsible for the differences in peanut allergy. Although there is clearly an inborn genetic predisposition toward food allergies, environmental factors, such as exposures to food proteins or other lifestyle exposures, account for a high proportion of the risk. You cannot change your parents or grandparents, but you may be able to change your environment. This notion has led to attempts at preventing allergy by manipulating the diet.

Is it possible to prevent food allergies and allergic disease through diet?

In short, the answer is "yes," but perhaps not in the way you might have guessed. Prevention of food allergies and other kinds does not seem to be related simply to whether allergenic foods are included in the diet.

Why is there a notion that avoiding allergenic foods might prevent food allergy?

A number of studies showed that infants who are fed a milk-based formula have a higher risk of atopic dermatitis or milk allergy compared with those who were breast fed. Studies performed over thirty years ago showed that infants fed a greater variety of solid foods earlier in life had an increased risk of having allergic eczema. These observations led to the idea that early exposure to whole proteins is a risk factor for allergy. Presumably, the young infant's immune or digestive system was ready for mother's milk, not whole proteins. An infant would not have been able to naturally drink from a cow's udder or to eat solid foods (unless the mother chewed them first and fed the spit to the baby, like a bird does for its chicks). Formula companies and baby food manufacturers have made it possible to give younger infants whole proteins, and this may be unnatural and a risk for allergy. These observations from decades ago, and the notion that infants are not ready for allergenic solids, resulted in the view that food allergies could be prevented by prolonged avoidance of common allergenic foods, such as milk, eggs, and peanuts.

Is avoiding allergenic foods by infants the right way to avoid food and other allergies?

Early studies suggested this may be the case and led to recommendations about prolonged avoidance of allergens as a strategy for avoiding food allergies. Not all these theories have stood the test of time, however. Some of the early observations may have been due to delayed allergy rather than prevention of allergy, and some of the early notions of a benefit to avoiding specific foods may be entirely wrong.

What is the difference between "preventing" and "delaying" allergy?
Prevention results from a change that permanently eliminates the allergy risk. Delaying an allergy, in contrast, means that some change in the diet resulted in not experiencing an allergic problem for some time, but that the allergy eventually occurs. This is an important distinction because attempts to prevent or delay childhood food allergies by avoidance of multiple foods risks nutritional deficiencies and affects quality of life. If doing so truly prevented an allergy, it might be worthwhile. However, if doing so merely delays allergy, it may not be worth altering the diet unless illness is observed first.

Why would an approach that prevents an allergy be better than one that delays an allergy?
Let's consider an example using a real study undertaken in the 1980s. One group of pregnant women with a family history of allergy avoided peanuts during pregnancy, used hypoallergenic formulas or breast fed while avoiding several allergens, and did not introduce milk until their babies were 1 year old, egg until age 2 years, and peanuts, tree nuts, and fish at 3 years. The comparison group did not follow these restrictions. In the first year or two, the infants from the group undertaking all these restrictions had significantly less eczema and milk allergy than the comparison group. However, at age 4 and 7 years, both groups had the same rate of milk allergy, eczema, asthma, and hay fever. Was it is worth undertaking all these restrictions in advance if they apparently did not have any permanent effect on preventing allergies? Perhaps a better strategy would be to wait and see whether any allergic problems developed and then alter the diet to address specific symptoms. This would lead to many fewer families undertaking troubling restrictions for no long-term benefit.

What strategies to prevent allergies have been studied?
Studies have addressed the following aspects of the mother's or infant's diet:

- The mother's diet during pregnancy
- Whether the infant is breast fed or formula fed

- The role of the mother's diet if breast feeding

- The type of formula used if formula feeding

- The timing of introduction of solid foods

- The timing of introduction of specific types of solid foods, especially eggs, milk, wheat, and peanuts

Additional studies have evaluated active forms of prevention that do not involve removing foods from the diet but instead give a treatment, such as probiotics (health-promoting bacteria), to attempt to reduce allergy risks.

PREGNANCY DIETS

Can a mother's diet during pregnancy protect her infant from allergy?

A handful of studies have specifically addressed the impact of peanut ingestion during pregnancy. Several small studies of highly allergic young children showed a relationship between a mother's ingestion of peanuts during pregnancy to peanut allergy. In contrast, several larger studies that did not focus on preselected allergic children did not show a relationship.

An analysis of the available studies of several foods concluded that maternal dietary exclusion does not appear to prevent allergy and carries a risk of fetal malnutrition. One study of over 2,500 German children focused on the maternal diet in the last four weeks of pregnancy and related the diet to eczema and "food sensitization" at the child's second birthday. The study found no relationship between the mothers' dietary intake of milk, eggs, or nuts and the allergy outcomes. Interestingly, maternal intake of margarine increased, and intake of fish decreased, the child's risk of eczema. This finding may be related to having "good fats" in the fish and "bad fats" in the margarine, which affect immune responses. It is notable that fish, a worrisome allergen, was protective of allergies.

Overall, there appears to be no strong evidence that the mother's restriction of allergens during pregnancy is preventive, although there is some controversy regarding peanuts.

**What do expert panels recommend regarding a mother's
diet during pregnancy for allergy prevention?**

A 2008 American Academy of Pediatrics report summa-
rized the overall findings that there was insufficient evidence to suggest
that maternal allergen avoidance during pregnancy significantly prevented allergies. A 2010 Food Allergy Expert Panel report concluded that
maternal allergen avoidance during pregnancy was not recommended.

**If there is controversy about the benefit of avoiding peanuts during pregnancy,
why do the experts not err on the side of saying avoid it?**

Expert panels have shied away from making recommendations when the
available evidence is unclear. The scientific community simply does not
know the best answer and would not want to give advice that may turn
out to be wrong or harmful.

What might an individual pregnant mother do about peanuts in her diet?

According to the current expert guidelines, there is no advice to avoid
foods such as peanuts. Individual families, however, can always use the
available information and their own experiences to make choices. Some
families have excluded peanuts from their home because of family members with peanut allergies. Some families find it easier to exclude an allergen to reduce the risk of accidentally ingesting it. In this situation, a
pregnant mother is already unlikely to ingest very much. For her it may
be sensible to follow a diet that is already in place. Statements from the
expert panels are not specifically recommending that peanut be increased
or excluded from the diet, so a pregnant mother should certainly feel at
liberty to manage her diet as she sees most reasonable.

BREAST FEEDING AND FORMULAS

Does breast feeding prevent allergy?

There are many reasons to breast feed, and exclusive breast feeding is encouraged for the first 4 to 6 months of infancy. In some studies of infants

at high risk of developing allergic diseases based on their family history, there is evidence that exclusive breast feeding for at least four months, compared with feeding cow's milk protein formula, reduces the risk of allergic eczema and cow's milk allergy at least in the first two years of life. Studies also generally show that exclusive breast feeding for at least three months protects against wheezing in early life. It is not clear, however, whether exclusive breast feeding has long-lasting effects on allergy prevention, and as more studies have been completed, there is more controversy as to whether breast feeding has a significant impact on preventing allergy.

Can a mother's diet during breast feeding prevent allergies?

Few studies address this question. It is known that a tiny amount of ingested protein can pass into breast milk. For some infants, that amount can induce allergic symptoms. It is not clear, however, whether this type of exposure, for most infants, is a potential means of causing an allergy or, perhaps, a natural way to teach the infant's immune system to accept various foods. If it is the latter, then a mother's diet may play a role in preventing allergy by including rather than excluding foods. Based on the very few available studies, allergen avoidance during breast feeding of an otherwise healthy infant does not appear to prevent allergic disease.

What do expert panels recommend regarding a mother's diet during lactation for allergy prevention?

A 2010 expert panel recommended against maternal allergen avoidance during lactation as a means to prevent food allergies. A 2008 American Academy of Pediatrics report had a similar conclusion, but recognized that limited studies showed reduction in allergic eczema when mothers avoided allergens in their diet. In summary, most of the evidence thus far does not support having a mother alter her diet while breast feeding as a means to prevent allergies.

What is the role of infant formulas for preventing food allergies?

Some infant formulas are derived from cow's milk or soybean. Typical formulas have whole proteins, similar to proteins in whole cow's milk or soy. Some infant formulas have predigested cow's milk proteins. This improves digestibility (partially hydrolyzed) or can make the formula safe for children with milk allergy (extensively hydrolyzed formula). There are also specialized formulas made from amino acids, the building blocks of proteins, and these are nonallergenic. No studies have found that infant formulas are superior to breast feeding for prevention of allergy.

Although breast milk is the best choice, are any infant formulas useful to prevent allergy?

Several studies suggest that specific predigested formulas, compared to standard whole cow's milk infant formulas, may delay or prevent allergic eczema. Not all formulas on the market have been specifically tested for the possibility of allergy prevention. A partially hydrolyzed whey-based formula (labeled as Good Start in the United States) appears to have a preventive effect, but possibly not as strong an effect as the extensively hydrolyzed formulas. Although studies are limited, soy formulas do not appear to provide protection compared with the whole cow's milk formulas. Various additional formulas have not yet been studied with regard to prevention, including ones made from mixtures of amino acids or various digests of milk.

What is the current approach to infant breast feeding or formula feeding to prevent allergies?

In summary, experts recommend exclusive breast feeding for the first 4 to 6 months of life. For infants with at least one parent or sibling with a documented allergy, who cannot be breast fed, or who need supplementation in the first months of life, the hypoallergenic or possibly less allergenic types of formula described above may reduce the risk of eczema and possibly milk allergy.

Is it better to exclusively breast feed or formula feed with a "prevention formula" even longer than 4 to 6 months?

Although the idea of "more is better" may apply, it has not been studied. The American Academy of Pediatrics report in 2008 concluded that there is not enough evidence to know if any dietary intervention has a protective effect after the age of 4 to 6 months. An infant is developmentally ready for solids in this time frame, and although breast feeding should continue, prolonging exclusive breast feeding has not been studied.

INTRODUCING SOLID FOODS

When should a baby eat solid foods?

The timing of introducing solid foods is partly related to the length of exclusive breast feeding, which is recommended for at least 4 to 6 months. Solids cannot be started until an infant has the developmental ability to swallow them. There is currently no convincing evidence that delaying solids, including potentially allergenic ones, for prolonged periods beyond 4 months of age has an impact on outcomes of allergic diseases.

What would be a possible exception to allowing an unrestricted diet for an infant who is prone to allergies?

If an infant is already showing signs of allergy, there may be additional potential allergens that could trigger reactions if offered. For example, an infant who already showed evidence of milk allergy is at increased risk of having egg or peanut allergy. In this situation, you should discuss additional allergen introductions with your doctor. For an infant who is otherwise well, there is a lack of evidence that waiting longer is protective.

What is the correct order for food introduction?

There is a tradition in the United States about introducing grains followed by vegetables and then fruits. This progression is not related to allergy. Many physicians recommend waiting several days between trying different foods because of concerns about allergy or intolerance, but this is also a traditional approach rather than one based on any specific studies. Various cultures introduce different foods in different sequences. Foods that are more difficult for an infant to safely ingest, such as choking hazards like pieces of meat, nuts, and so forth, by default must be introduced later, when a baby is able to manage them without choking.

CURRENT RECOMMENDATIONS

How have the recommendations about allergy prevention through diet changed over time?

In 2000, the American Academy of Pediatrics recommended that mothers with a family history of allergy consider avoiding peanuts during pregnancy and allergenic foods during lactation, then not introduce milk until age 1 year, egg until age 2, and peanuts, tree nuts, and fish until age 3. The experts explained that these recommendations were not based on specific evidence from studies, but that they seemed reasonable given the state of knowledge at the time. All these recommendations were overturned in 2008. The committee on toxicology in the UK recommended similar restrictions on peanuts around the same time but has also withdrawn those recommendations. Various other expert panels from Europe and other countries never dictated specific allergen avoidance for the mother or infant.

Why did recommendations about dietary restrictions to prevent allergy change?

Medical societies and expert panels have taken the approach of avoiding recommendations unless there is reasonable evidence. Over the years, since the American Academy of Pediatrics made recommendations in 2000, studies have raised questions about the effectiveness of prolonged avoidance of allergens such as milk, eggs, wheat, and peanut. For example, several large studies showed an increased risk of milk, egg, and wheat allergy or allergic eczema among children who waited longer to have these foods added to their diet.

It was also observed that Jewish children in the UK have a 10 times higher rate of peanut allergy compared with Jewish children in Israel. One difference between these countries is that the Israeli children eat peanut snacks in the first year of life while the children in the UK generally do not eat peanuts until well after a year. These studies cast doubt on a preventive effect of waiting prolonged periods to introduce allergens into the diet, and they were responsible, in part, for withdrawal of prior recommendations.

Why might waiting longer to introduce foods have resulted in a stronger risk for food allergy?

If these studies suggesting that prolonged avoidance increases allergy risks are correct (there is some controversy; see "Delving Deeper" near the end of this chapter), there are several theories as to why. Although infants under about 4 months are not physically, or probably immunologically, ready to ingest solid foods or whole natural proteins (their bodies are designed to be breast fed), after this age the immune system may be "ready" and may actually benefit from being exposed to the food orally so that the immune system learns to "accept" the foods. Another theory suggests that prolonged avoidance of eating an allergen may leave the infant's immune system more likely to become allergic through non-oral exposures to foods, such as through skin exposure.

What evidence is there that skin exposure to food allergens might increase the risk of food allergy?

So far, only two studies, both from the UK, support this theory, and they both relate to peanuts. One study evaluated allergy-prone children and found that those who developed peanut allergies were more likely to have lived in homes where more peanuts were consumed (while the infant was generally avoiding eating it). The infants who had eaten peanuts earlier appeared to have more protection from developing peanut allergies than those who did not, in the homes with high peanut consumption. Another study suggested that infants who had their skin rashes treated with peanut-containing skin creams had a higher risk of peanut allergy (these creams are not generally used in the United States). Thus, these two studies suggest that allergy-prone infants with eczema may develop peanut allergies from household exposures, especially through rashy skin, and especially if they have not been eating peanut.

Should all infants be given allergens like peanuts and nuts earlier?

Traditionally in the United States, grains, fruits, and vegetables are the first solid foods. Foods selected for infants must be a consistency the infant can manage, so choking hazards such as nuts are not typically given early. Although the American Academy of Pediatrics recommendations from 2000 that suggested delayed introductions of milk, eggs, peanuts, nuts, and fish have since been revoked, there are no specific recommendations to introduce these allergenic foods "early" as first foods. In fact, if a child already had an allergic reaction to some foods, such as milk or egg, that child is at higher risk of already being allergic to other allergens. In this situation, discussion with an allergist is warranted before advancing the diet. For an otherwise healthy infant, however, there are no restrictions.

NONDIETARY ASPECTS OF PREVENTION

Aside from allergen-related diet restrictions, how else might one prevent allergies?

Most of the attention regarding allergy prevention has focused on removing allergenic foods from the diet. We now know that some of these past recommendations were likely incorrect and possibly counterproductive. Studies are under way to try to learn if there are other ways to prevent allergies, and these focus on identifying risk factors that could be modified, such as the following targets:

- *Obesity.* Obesity has been associated with an increased risk for allergies, although the relationship is unclear. Perhaps children with food allergies eat more calorically enriched foods or, more likely, since obesity is associated with a state of increased inflammation, this inflammation might bias the immune system toward allergy.

- *Vitamin D deficiency.* There is evidence that vitamin D deficiency may also increase risks. Dietary lack of vitamin D, or less sunlight (which allows our skin to produce vitamin D), may result in deficiency. Vitamin D is necessary for healthy immune responses.

- *Poor intake of healthy dietary fats.* As mentioned previously, a diet with immune system–promoting fats from fish rather than fats from margarine may be beneficial. A balanced healthy diet and lifestyle is likely an important aspect of prevention.

- *Hygiene.* The increasing rate of allergy may be associated with improved hygiene, leading to misfiring of the immune system. To address the possibility that a lack of exposure to germs is at fault, research has turned to providing exposure to health-promoting bacteria—probiotics.

Do probiotics prevent allergies?

Probiotics are live bacteria thought to have health-promoting effects. Prebiotics are food substances that help our bodies maintain these health-promoting bacteria. Increasingly, studies are evaluating the use of prebiotics and probiotics for prevention of allergic disease. There are many different types of probiotic bacteria, and their effects may vary. Some studies have suggested that early use of probiotics may reduce the risk of allergic eczema. Curiously, some of the studies showing this benefit also found possible increase in positive allergy tests to foods, although the numbers of children with this finding were quite small. Concerns regarding probiotics include the possibility of having an infection from them or having a reaction to milk contamination, because many of them are grown in milk. Nonetheless, this is a promising area of investigation that has shown some positive results in reducing the risk of allergy. Talk to your doctor about whether this is an option for you.

If my child has allergies, can I do something to prevent new ones?

Unfortunately, children who develop a food allergy or any allergic disease are at risk for developing others. The "allergic march" refers to the observation that young children with allergic eczema or food allergies are at increased risk to "march on" to develop allergic asthma and hay fever. Although research is under way, we currently do not have any proven means to reduce the risk aside from those mentioned previously.

What is the risk that a child with food allergies and eczema will develop asthma?

Over 50%.

How can an adult with food allergies avoid getting new ones?

We do not have any sure ways to avoid new food allergies. Studies suggest that treatment of the pollen allergy with immunotherapy (allergy shots) may help some people to reduce symptoms from the related fruits or vegetables (oral allergy syndrome). Immunotherapy is usually suggested when hay fever is not responding well to medications such as antihistamines, medicated nose sprays, and eye drops. For persons undergoing immunotherapy, an added benefit may be reduced symptoms from the foods that are related to pollens. Not all studies support this observation, but it may be an extra benefit of having pollen immunotherapy for some people. Presumably this treatment would prevent additional related fruits or vegetables from becoming problematic, but this is unproved.

Delving Deeper:
DIFFICULTIES IN STUDYING ALLERGY PREVENTION

What are the limitations of studies on allergy prevention?

Most of the studies on risks and potential prevention of allergies are not designed as experiments; rather, researchers watch behaviors and look for outcomes. Unfortunately, these types of nonexperimental studies carry many biases. For example, a family that perceives eggs to be a risk factor for allergy in their allergy-prone family may purposely delay giving eggs. Their child, who is already at risk for allergy, may well develop an allergy. Meanwhile, children at low allergy risk who are not avoiding eggs will usually be fine. A study that includes these families may wrongly conclude that delaying eggs "caused" the allergy when really it was a risk of allergy that caused delayed introduction of eggs! These limitations have led to designing experimental studies to evaluate these issues without bias.

The LEAP study (Learning Early About Peanut allergy) randomly assigns "at risk" children to eat peanuts early or to delay. The LEAP study is avoiding potential bias by assigning the timing of peanut introduction. We hope this study and others will begin to answer the questions about timing in the introduction of allergenic foods.

Also of Interest:
INSIGHTS ON PREVENTION FROM WORLDWIDE OBSERVATIONS

Can we learn anything about prevention from worldwide differences in allergy rates?

Peanut allergy is less common in China and Africa where peanuts are boiled or fried, and more common in the United States, Canada, Australia, and other countries, where peanuts are typically dry roasted. It may be that dry roasting peanuts alters the proteins in a way that could increase their ability to trigger allergy. Another theory suggests that the oily base of peanut butter may further promote an adverse immune response. Perhaps we should stop using roasted peanut products?

This theory about roasted peanuts has limitations because worldwide allergy rates may vary for other reasons. In the study comparing peanut allergies in Jewish children in the UK to those in Israel, described earlier in this chapter, both groups were exposed to roasted forms of peanuts, but the Israeli children, who had one-tenth the rate of peanut allergies, generally ingested this food before age 1, compared with after age 2 or 3 in the UK. Thus, timing of ingestion may be the more important factor, rather than roasting, although there may be other differences between these countries that could explain the different peanut allergy rates. For example, allergies to foods other than peanut are also less common in nonwesternized countries. Differences in industrialization within the same country appear to have an effect as well. Rural areas of China have fewer food allergies and allergic diseases than urbanized areas. Therefore, the hygiene hypothesis may be a significant component of these observed worldwide differences.

Scientists are looking to maintain the advantages but avoid the risks of our modern lifestyle. Active approaches include studies of health-promoting bacteria (probiotics), the use of harmless parasites (to keep the allergy arm of the immune system occupied), and the timing of food introduction. Studies continue to address the potential risks of food processing, the use of medications, how obesity may promote allergy, vitamin or other nutrient deficiencies, and many other factors that may provide insight into the allergy "epidemic" and identify ways to prevent allergies to food and other substances.

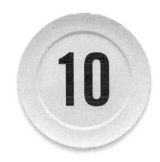

Will There Be a **CURE** or **BETTER TREATMENT** of Food Allergy?

This chapter answers your questions about treatments of food allergy that may be available in the near future and about food allergy research in general.

GENERAL QUESTIONS ABOUT FOOD ALLERGY RESEARCH

What are the goals of research in food allergy?

There are many research goals, such as determining how many people are affected, risk factors, prevention strategies, better ways to diagnose and, of course, better treatments. Additional areas include how to better educate people about managing their food allergies and improving quality of life. This chapter focuses on research for better treatments and cures.

What types of research currently address treatment of food allergies?

There are two broad categories of research: studies done in the laboratory and studies done in people. Both types are active. There are two types of approaches to treatments as well. One type is directed toward a particular food, such as peanuts or eggs, and would work only for that specific food, and another approach is to find a therapy to work for any food allergy.

What are clinical trials?

Clinical trials are ones performed in people to see if a therapy is safe and effective.

What are the prospects for future therapies to treat food allergies?

The future looks bright. Many ideas are being evaluated in the laboratory, and several clinical trials are evaluating various treatment options.

Who funds research on food allergies?

Research studies are funded in many ways. Your tax dollars may pay for studies through grants from the National Institutes of Health. Donations directly to researchers or through organizations that raise money for research are another source of funds. Pharmaceutical companies also fund research studies. Still, a major hindrance to progress is the lack of funding to allow the many good ideas for laboratory and clinical studies to progress.

Who regulates or supervises research on food allergies?

Research studies are regulated or supervised in various ways. If a study involves animals, institutional committees monitor the animals' welfare. When studies involve people, review boards address the safety and the scientific background of the study. Clinical studies often require an ongoing review board not associated with the study to evaluate safety and progress. Additionally, if the study involves a drug or a medical device, there is an additional review by the Food and Drug Administration. In some cases, even more additional committees that address safety and scientific value will review a study, depending on the treatment being performed and the source of funding. The review process includes various experts and laypersons who ensure that the study is done safely, for good reasons, and that it is sensitive to participants who may be especially vulnerable, such as children.

How are research advances in food allergies reported?

Researchers generally publish their findings in research journals. The reports undergo evaluation by experts before being published. Preliminary reports are often communicated at scientific meetings. The general public usually hears about research advances through the media. It can be confusing to know if the research result is significant or immediately applicable. Talk to your allergist if you believe you might benefit from some new finding.

How do scientists interpret their food allergy research results?

Carefully! It can be difficult to come to conclusions if a study suffers from limitations, and most studies are not perfect. For example, on a hot day the pavement is hot and more people sweat. Is the hot pavement causing them to sweat? Will cooling the pavement reduce sweating? It may appear that way unless one considers that the sun was responsible for overheating both the person and the pavement. Many research studies rely on situations that are not controllable, for example, a mother's choice to breast feed her infant. If a large group of mothers believed that breast feeding reduces allergic rashes and continued to breast feed when they saw any rash, then it could seem that breast feeding actually causes rashes. The best type of studies randomize people to a type of treatment and have a "fake" treatment (a placebo) so that those on a treatment and the people evaluating them do not know who is on the therapy being tested.

When does a research result cause a change in food allergy management?

Most research studies add small pieces to a larger puzzle. As evidence mounts, it is easier for people to be confident that the results are true and that a treatment or approach may be worthwhile. Often, the research on a particular topic from several different studies is analyzed together to ensure that the overall results from numerous studies are truly identifying a benefit (an approach called a meta-analysis). The available information is also evaluated by experts, often government agencies, and others to recommend changes in practice. Sometimes, the evidence remains unclear and experts must choose whether to recommend a specific approach. Additionally, your own doctor might consider the available evidence and your specific circumstances to make decisions. For a new approach or treatment to be widely available and accepted, as well as covered by insurance, the approach typically has to go through extensive phases of study to understand the risks and benefits as well as the effectiveness (and to prove the effectiveness).

What types of basic science research are under way for food allergies?
Many laboratory studies evaluate the basic mechanisms underlying food allergies, trying to understand how and why the immune system "attacks" foods as well as various means that might interrupt or reverse that process.

What are "translational" studies of food allergy?
Translational research refers to moving laboratory discoveries into people. Initial studies done at the laboratory bench are "translated" into treatments that are tried in people.

What types of clinical studies are under way to treat food allergies?
The two main types are those that are designed to treat an allergy to any food, and those that are focused on the treatment of a specific food (for example, just milk or just peanut).

What are examples of food allergy treatments that are not specific to particular foods?
Examples include anti-IgE therapy, remedies based on traditional Chinese medicine, and treatments that block immune responses.

What are examples of food allergy treatments that are specific to particular foods?
Examples include giving a person the food to which they are allergic, or a modified form of that food, in gradually increasing amounts (immunotherapy).

How do I keep abreast of what studies are under way and what progress has been made in food allergy therapy?
This is a fast-moving area, and although this chapter gives updates and insights on current treatments, you will need to talk to your doctor about what is currently available. There are many additional resources (see chapter 11) to learn about research progress.

Which food allergy treatment under study is most likely to work in the long run?
We do not know which treatment will win out as safest and most effective.
It is promising that numerous therapies are being tested. A particular
therapy may be beneficial for some people and not others, and treatments
may need to be individualized.

APPROACHES TO TREAT ANY TYPE OF FOOD ALLERGY

What is anti-IgE therapy for food allergies?
Most severe food allergies with a rapid onset of symptoms are triggered
by the body producing IgE. This treatment is an injected protein that essentially ties up and inactivates the IgE. The therapy has been in use for
chronic allergic asthma that has not responded well to other therapies.
The theory behind the treatment is that inactivating the body's IgE will
prevent allergic reactions to any food.

What have studies shown for using anti-IgE for food allergies?
The studies have so far shown that people on this type of therapy can
generally ingest more of the food than when they are not treated. Not all
people experience an improvement, however, and the degree of improvement varies.

What are potential advantages of anti-IgE therapy for food allergies?
The fact that the treatment can address any food allergy is a great advantage. Being able to increase the threshold where a person reacts could
reduce the danger of small exposures for sensitive people.

What are potential problems with anti-IgE therapy for food allergies?
There are several. Some people make so much IgE that the treatment cannot overcome it and cannot be used at all. The treatment itself sometimes
causes an allergic reaction. For those who had some benefit, the therapy
does not seem to completely block allergic reactions in many.

What is the status of anti-IgE therapy for food allergy?

At the time of this writing, more studies were being done to better characterize the effectiveness and safety of this approach.

What are Chinese herbal remedies for food allergy?

Traditional Chinese medicine has been used for centuries to treat many conditions, but food allergy was not a strong concern in the past. Dr. Xiu-Min Li at the Jaffe Food Allergy Institute at Mount Sinai, New York, where I work, developed a remedy selecting components from the traditional medicine formulary, based on various symptoms one develops from food allergy. She found the therapy to be effective in mice that were allergic. The treatment has mostly been evaluated in mice with peanut allergy but also appears effective for other foods.

What types of food allergies could be treated by Chinese herbal remedies?

Any. The therapy is not designed for a specific food or foods.

What is the status of research using Chinese herbal remedies for food allergy?

In mice, the therapy allows them to eat the food to which they were allergic well beyond the end of a treatment period. When the allergy begins to recur, retreatment protects the mice again. The therapy is made of many different components, and it is important to ensure the components are the same with each batch, so much care is taken in growing and processing the ingredients. Studies are focusing on determining the most crucial ingredients so they can be isolated for a therapy. In the meantime, the treatment dose requires a large number of pills each day. Initial studies have supported the safety of the therapy, but research is now being done to see if the treatment helps people, not just mice.

What are probiotics, prebiotics, and synbiotics?

Probiotics are live microorganisms that, when administered in adequate amounts, confer a health benefit. Prebiotics are nutrients that help the healthy bacteria grow and survive, and "synbiotics" refers to the use of both at the same time.

How might probiotics, prebiotics, and synbiotics treat food allergies?

The hygiene hypothesis of allergy suggests that our clean living leaves our immune system "looking for a fight," and without plenty of germs, it is more likely to attack harmless proteins in foods. By providing health-promoting bacteria, researchers hope the immune system will become better balanced and less likely to attack innocent proteins.

What is the status of research on probiotics, prebiotics, and synbiotics for food allergy?

Regarding treatment, the results have been poor. Most studies so far have not shown an effect, but research is ongoing. See chapter 9 for the role of these treatments for prevention.

What are parasites, specifically TSO, and what do they have to do with food allergy treatment?

TSO is short for *Trichuris suis* ova (eggs), a type of parasite (worm) egg that is live but cannot live long term in people (they can live in pigs). Antiallergy treatment with this parasite is based on the idea that the immune system's allergic responses involve the same cells and proteins used to fight parasites. Additionally, people living in parasitized regions of the globe tend to have fewer allergies. Thus, treatment with TSO is based on reasoning that having parasites may promote less allergy and that using a parasite that is generally "safe" is a useful strategy. However, it also could be argued that this type of treatment might "rev up" an existing allergy .

How might TSO treat food allergies?

This is not clear and has not been researched sufficiently yet.

What is the status of research on parasites and TSO for food allergy?

There was a supportive study on its use in an inflammatory bowel disease called Crohn disease, but there are limited studies in allergy. One study of hay fever did not show a benefit, and the people treated had side effects of stomach pain and diarrhea.

APPROACHES TO TREAT ALLERGIES TO SPECIFIC FOODS

Why are there allergy shots for pollen and environmental allergies but not food allergies?

"Allergy shots," or immunotherapy using injections, are effective for pollen allergies and allergies to stinging insects. They seem to work by reeducating the immune system not to "attack" the injected proteins by exposing a person to small and increasing amounts over weeks and months. In the 1980s, studies were begun using peanuts for injections. The treatment made it possible for the participants to eat a larger amount of peanuts, but the side effects of the treatment were too strong; people had allergic reactions, sometimes severe ones, to the allergy shots, and the strategy was abandoned.

What are the different strategies for immunotherapy or allergy shots for food allergies?

The primary approach is to expose the immune system to the food proteins without triggering allergic reactions. Different strategies to do this include altering the proteins to make them less potent for triggering a reaction and more capable of promoting protective responses, or giving the proteins in a manner other than through an injection, for example, by mouth, so that severe reactions to the treatment are less likely. Proteins can be engineered without parts that are more potent, chopped into smaller pieces that are less allergenic, or treated in ways that alter their structure. The treatment can also include proteins or other compounds that promote nonallergic reactions and target the treatment to the immune system in a way that promotes treatment.

What is the status of research on various modified vaccines for food allergies?

A treatment using modified peanut allergens, engineered to have less potency, worked well in mice with peanut allergy. However, when used in a safety study in people, there were still allergic reactions from the treatment. This therapy will need to be re-evaluated, perhaps to give a lower dose or to further alter the peanut proteins.

What are oral and sublingual immunotherapies?

Oral or sublingual immunotherapies involve gradually giving the allergic food by mouth or as an extract under the tongue. Typically, a dose is given under medical supervision, and then the dose is continued daily at home until a slightly higher dose is given under medical supervision. The gradual increases in dosing are usually stopped when a targeted daily dose is reached. This strategy has been described in the literature for many decades. *But do not try this at home! Reactions can occur!*

What is the status of treatment using sublingual immunotherapy for food allergies?

The studies thus far have been promising in that allergic reactions to the therapy are generally mild and uncommon, and persons on the treatment experience an increased threshold compared to those treated with placebo. However, the improvement has generally not been strong enough for most people to eat regular servings of the food.

What is the status of treatment using oral immunotherapy for food allergies?

This therapy has been the most frequently tested in the last ten years. Studies are ongoing to try to determine if the treatment can "cure" an allergy or only improve the amount of a food that can be ingested while on treatment.

What are the advantages of oral or sublingual immunotherapy for food allergies?

This approach appears to carry less risk than injection immunotherapy with a food. The treatment is painless and convenient.

What are the disadvantages of oral or sublingual immunotherapy for food allergies?

Some people have allergic reactions to the doses that are given as treatment. Sometimes epinephrine is needed. Furthermore, the treatment is only effective for the food that is being targeted.

What are the advantages or disadvantages of oral versus sublingual immunotherapy for food allergies?

From studies available thus far, it appears that the oral route of treatment, compared to the sublingual, is more effective but also more likely to cause allergic reactions.

What are some of the successes in oral immunotherapy for food allergies?

Most people treated with this approach are able to increase the amount of the food they can ingest.

What are some of the pitfalls in oral immunotherapy for food allergies?

In most studies, about 20% cannot tolerate the dosing and must abandon therapy. Those who can continue treatment may experience allergic reactions to the daily dose that is taken. Sometimes there are reactions to previously tolerated daily doses. This appears to occur more often if the person contracts an illness, is exercising, or is menstruating.

Does oral immunotherapy or sublingual immunotherapy permanently cure a food allergy or only change how much food can be eaten while the person is taking treatment?

As mentioned previously, the treatment usually allows a person to ingest more of the allergen, a result called "desensitization." It remains under investigation whether this approach to treatment can be a "cure," meaning that the allergy is gone even when the daily dosing is ceased, a result called permanent "tolerance."

So far, studies appear to show that if doses are missed, there can be a loss of treatment effect such that a dose previously taken without symptoms may induce reactions. This has occurred after even brief periods of not treating (for example, a few days). Therefore, it appears that desensitization can occur without tolerance.

Most studies have not compared the results of longer periods (years) of treatment, which may induce more permanent changes.

Is oral or sublingual immunotherapy for food allergy an approved treatment?

At the time of this writing, no. Larger trials are needed and being planned prior to seeking FDA approval.

Can I find a physician who will use oral or sublingual immunotherapy for food allergy treatment?
You may be able to because doctors may use an approach without approval. Caution is advised. Most experts believe that this should not be done until FDA approval is granted.

How will treatments such as oral or sublingual immunotherapy for food allergies become approved?
Larger studies must prove acceptable safety and effectiveness. If the treatment does not cause a permanent cure, it will be crucial to know who will most likely benefit, how much, and with what risks. A major concern to be addressed is that an individual may lose the treatment effect and become allergic if he or she does not take a daily dose of the food or stops eating the food for a period.

If a person with milk or egg allergies can tolerate eating these foods when they are baked into breads or muffins, does eating these foods help to treat these allergies?
As discussed in chapter 6, about 70% to 80% of children with allergy to whole forms of milk or eggs (scrambled eggs, French toast, cheese, ice cream, and so on) can tolerate baked goods with these ingredients. For those who do, it is not entirely clear whether this speeds, hinders, or has no impact on recovery from the allergy. Preliminary studies of milk and eggs have suggested that the milk or egg-allergic children who tolerate these extensively heated foods show immune changes that are similar to people treated with oral or sublingual immunotherapy and that this may speed recovery compared with strict avoidance.

What is epicutaneous (on the skin) immunotherapy for food allergy?
Another approach to immunotherapy is to place the food on the skin for prolonged periods in a way that allows absorption. The theory is that immune cells in the skin may promote a nonallergic response to the food over time.

What are advantages of epicutaneous immunotherapy for food allergy?

A primary advantage is safety because foods placed on the skin are unlikely to trigger anaphylaxis, although rashes are possible.

What progress has been made in epicutaneous immunotherapy for food allergies?

Preliminary studies on milk allergy showed a trend toward increasing the amount of milk that is tolerated. Additional studies on milk and peanuts are ongoing.

Is there a potential for combining therapies?

Yes. For example, low doses of a food given sublingually may be a starting point for using larger doses in oral immunotherapy. Also, using anti-IgE therapy prior to and while initially increasing doses of oral immunotherapy may potentially reduce side effects and improve the effectiveness of the treatment.

What is the progress in using immunotherapy and anti-IgE treatment at the same time for food allergies?

Initial studies have been promising in perhaps reducing, although not eliminating, the reactions to dosing.

What additional treatments are being evaluated to treat food allergies?

Please see chapter 11 to learn more about how to access information on current studies. A number of novel therapies that were promising in preclinical studies may be ready for trials in people. Some possibilities include "peptides" that represent chopped up food allergens, allergens attached to or targeted to immune cells that promote healthy immune responses, and drugs that target allergy cells responsible for the allergic symptoms, attempting to cripple them from becoming activated and releasing their chemicals.

TREATMENTS OF SPECIFIC FOOD-ALLERGIC DISEASES

What treatments are being evaluated for eosinophilic esophagitis?

Current treatments include dietary avoidance of allergens and use of steroids. New therapies are targeting the cells and chemicals that direct the allergic inflammation. See chapter 5 for more information about this illness and its treatment.

What treatments are being evaluated to treat anaphylaxis?

New forms of epinephrine autoinjectors are being considered. Drugs and other treatment to block the cells and chemicals that cause the symptoms are being analyzed.

What treatments are being evaluated to treat oral allergy syndrome?

Allergen immunotherapy (allergy shots) and other treatments of pollen allergy may have the useful additional benefit of also reducing or eliminating symptoms from the food proteins that are similar to the pollen proteins.

What treatments are being tested for food protein–induced enterocolitis syndrome?

Currently, the main therapy is food avoidance. Studies are attempting to determine the cells and immune responses that are causing these reactions so that targets for treatments can be found. It is not currently known whether treatments for IgE-mediated allergy, such as oral immunotherapy, would help enterocolitis syndrome.

UNPROVEN TREATMENTS

What food allergy treatments are unproved?

Throughout this book, various approaches to treatment are discussed that remain under study and may be considered "unproved" or perhaps only partly proved. This is somewhat a semantic concern. For example, oral immunotherapy has been shown to alter the threshold of reactivity to foods for many people, and so in one way it is "proved" to work, and yet more needs to be done to determine if the effects can be long-lasting, to minimize side effects, and so forth. So oral immunotherapy could be considered partly unproved. Other treatments, however, would be considered inappropriate because they are unproved or even disproved and not based on firm evidence.

What food allergy treatments would be considered inappropriate?

Traditional allergists consider several approaches used today to be inappropriate. These include acupressure, chiropractic manipulation, provocation-neutralization therapy, rotation diets, orthomolecular therapy, mercury amalgam removal, urine autoinjection, laser therapy, antifungal therapy, and immune system–boosting elimination diets.

What is provocation-neutralization therapy?

This treatment, also discussed in chapter 3, relies on diagnosing food allergies by provoking symptoms using dilutions of the allergen and then treating them by using a weaker "neutralizing" dose. The treatment has been disproved in well-designed studies.

What are rotation diets?

The general theory is that there may be foods in the diet causing "symptoms," and by rotating what is eaten every four or five days, the body is not exposed to large amounts of any particular problematic food. Additionally, the theory is that reducing continued exposure to particular foods would reduce the chance of developing problems with them. This theory runs counter to many proven aspects of food allergy; for example, if a food is an allergen for a person, symptoms will arise whenever the food is eaten. It is also counter to the observation that maintaining exposure to a food may actually reduce the chance of allergy in some cases.

What is orthomolecular therapy?

This treatment approach, used infrequently for food allergy but often for a variety of maladies, relies on giving large doses of various vitamins, supplements, and antioxidants in response to measurement of vitamins in the serum. There are no controlled studies of this approach, and there are dangers of overdosing vitamins.

What is mercury amalgam removal?

There is a theory that silver-mercury amalgam used in dental fillings may cause sensitivity that results in various maladies and symptoms. This theory remains unproved, so removal of the fillings as a treatment is unproved.

What is urine autoinjection?

Based on observations in the 1930s that the urine of some allergic people injected into their own skin caused a response but that their urine injected into another person did not, some practitioners began to inject urine as a treatment of various illnesses (allergies, stomach complaints, jaundice, and so forth). There were never any good studies on the effectiveness, and this treatment could actually promote adverse immune responses against the body's own proteins. Professional organizations have warned against this practice as unproved, without scientific basis, and potentially dangerous.

What is laser therapy?

The laser method purportedly uses a biofeedback machine to simulate and test reactions to thousands of allergens before a laser is used to stimulate the nervous system. No studies support the claim that this technology cures allergies. Legislation to outlaw its use has been submitted. Some advertise that the approach is FDA approved, which is not accurate.

What is antifungal therapy?

There is a theory that yeast in the body, *Candida*, is responsible for a "yeast hypersensitivity syndrome" in which overgrowth results in inflammation and toxins. The symptoms attributed to this include fatigue, heartburn, bloating, diarrhea, constipation, depression, and memory problems. However, *Candida* and other fungi are normal inhabitants of the body, and there is no routine diagnostic approach to an overgrowth or toxic effect. Treatments have included various diets and antifungal therapies. A scientific basis for a syndrome has never been established. One well-controlled study did not show improvement in general symptoms of fatigue or depression from treatments against the fungus.

What are immune system–boosting elimination diets?

Through combinations of testing, using traditional or alternative and unproved methods, numerous foods are eliminated from the diet to treat presumed "multiple food allergy" with the notion that doing so may improve the immune system. Often, the person is given various dietary supplements. There is no evidence that removal of multiple foods improves immune function, and it may actually risk problems from malnutrition.

PARTICIPATING IN FOOD ALLERGY RESEARCH

What is it like to participate in food allergy clinical trials?

Most clinical trials of food allergy involve a screening visit to ensure the participant is otherwise generally healthy and qualifies for the study. An initial feeding test is often used to determine how much food can be consumed before symptoms occur. Next, treatment is started (randomized, like a coin toss, to receive the therapy being tested or placebo), and after some period another feeding test is performed to check for effectiveness, comparing the treatment to placebo. During the entire study, the participant keeps in close contact with the study investigators and staff.

Should I participate in clinical trials for food allergy?

This is a personal decision. If people did not participate, however, we would never learn whether a treatment works, and no progress would be made. In fact, recruitment of participants into research studies, for all treatments, not just food allergy, is a major hurdle that results in delays in moving treatments forward or in learning which ones to abandon. If a clinical trial is not for you, you can still contribute to food allergy research by participating in studies that involve only questionnaires or a blood sample, through donations toward research, or through advocacy.

What are the advantages of participating in clinical trials for food allergy?

The primary advantage is to help determine if a particular approach is viable for treating food allergy. There is a potential benefit for the participant to experience some improvement in the allergy, but if this were a definite benefit, there would be no need for a study! Participants often feel empowered because they are doing something to help themselves and others who are suffering with food allergies (whether or not the treatment under study is proved effective).

What are the disadvantages of participating in clinical trials for food allergy?

There are typically general risks associated with trying a new therapy because there may be side effects. These would be described in detail and would depend on the approach and type of study. Other disadvantages are related to time commitments and discomfort (such as blood tests). These issues vary greatly among studies. Most treatment trials are mimicking what would be done should the therapy prove to be effective. Thus, the number of visits is not much different from what would be done if the therapy became routine clinical practice.

What is done to ensure safety if I participate in clinical trials for food allergy?

Many things. Investigators are likely to explain that they would not enroll people into a trial unless they felt they would have themselves or their own family members participate as well. As described earlier in this chapter, the study procedures are evaluated by external reviewers, often through numerous different regulators. Each procedure is performed under the appropriate supervision to ensure safety. Any adverse effects are monitored and evaluated. Privacy is as carefully protected as is possible under law. A participant is always free to leave a study. In fact, if the investigators are concerned about a participant's safety, they can remove the person from the study, even if the participant wanted to continue.

How are people selected for clinical trials of food allergy?

The entry criteria for a study typically addresses the illness being studied. For example, a study of a treatment for milk allergy requires people with milk allergy. Depending on several factors, an age range may be specified.

Why are some people excluded from clinical trials of food allergy?

All studies establish criteria that exclude participants. Sometimes the exclusions have to do with the treatment being used. For example, a person who makes too much or no IgE may not qualify for a study of an anti-IgE therapy. Often, people cannot participate if they are on treatments that might interfere with evaluating the response to the therapy being tested. Many of the exclusions are for safety reasons; for example, a person with significant medical problems other than food allergy is not likely to be a good candidate because there could be added risks due to those health issues. The same is true for having severe, poorly controlled asthma.

Why are specific age groups included in individual studies for food allergy treatments?

When treatments are initially trialed, healthy adults may be the first to be tested just to learn how the body manages the treatment. As therapies are tested further, adults, teenagers, or children over age 12 might be tested initially before trying the therapy on younger children—again, to ensure safety. Also, the older participants are better able to discuss any side effects.

Should I be concerned about the oral food challenges that are part of food allergy trials?

Oral food challenges are discussed in detail in chapter 3. When they are performed in research studies, the risk of having symptoms is greater because, unlike diagnostic tests, the person being tested is assumed to be allergic. Therefore, starting doses and timing of doses is likely to be different in research studies. Still, the purpose of the feeding test is to determine how much of the food triggers symptoms; the purpose is *not to cause a severe reaction*. The feeding is stopped when a reaction is evident. The most common symptoms are skin and gut symptoms. The studies are always performed under medical supervision. Discuss any concerns with your study doctor.

What if I am randomly assigned to the placebo in a food allergy clinical trial?
Potential research participants may feel that they do not want to participate because they do not want to be randomized to receive the placebo. There are many reasons this should not be a concern:

- The study is not likely to be valid if there is no placebo comparison. In a study of anti-IgE therapy, the placebo group was able to eat three times more peanuts after therapy (placebo therapy). This sounds pretty good, but any ineffective treatment could have this placebo effect. If you participate in a study without a placebo group, the chance that the study will provide strong evidence for or against the new therapy is diminished, and your commitment may not have been as worthwhile in finding an answer.

- If the therapy does work, and you were in the placebo group, you will still have access, eventually, to a useful treatment.

- If the therapy had unanticipated side effects, you will have avoided them.

How do I find out about clinical trials and food allergy?
There are many sources (see chapter 11). In the United States, an excellent resource is www.clinicaltrials.gov, where you can search for clinical trials using terms that describe what you are looking for (for example, milk allergy).

How do I stay informed about new treatments for food allergy?
Get on a mailing list of any nearby research centers, join lay organizations and support groups, and look at the websites that act as clearinghouses for trials and for other types of food allergy research.

How do I become an advocate for food allergy research?
Join a group! See the resources in chapter 11.

Delving Deeper:
CHINESE HERBAL THERAPIES

How did the Chinese herbal remedy make its way to clinical trials?

Dr. Xiu-Min Li, mentioned above, studied traditional Chinese medicine and brought her knowledge to the laboratory. She and her team developed mouse "models" of food allergy and tested the concoction of remedies until an effective formulation was found. She could not at first convince the National Institutes of Health (NIH) to support her work, and her initial studies were supported by grants raised through donations to the Food Allergy Initiative (FAI), a nonprofit organization based in New York. With her promising results in mice, and with the establishment of the National Center for Complementary and Alternative Medicine, an arm of the NIH, she eventually obtained funds to further her studies.

The mice were noted to be virtually cured of peanut allergy for prolonged periods after an initial treatment and were responsive to retreatment when their protection waned. Studies showed that the effect was not like those seen from known antiallergy drugs, but there were changes in the immune response. It was also clear that removal of some components reduced the effectiveness, making the formulation complex and difficult to distill into a palatable treatment. Still, a final formulation was made and a starting dose mimicking what the mice were given was developed (ten small pills three times each day). Given the treatment safety in mice, the government and FAI supported a study in which the formula was ingested for a week and then six months, also without safety concerns, allowing the treatment to be tested in a trial to see if it works in people, not just mice. Meanwhile, Dr. Li and her team are trying to identify active ingredients to focus on a more specific therapy.

Also of Interest:
WHY HAS RESEARCH BEEN SO SLOW?

Why has progress been so slow in food allergy immunotherapy?

A report going back to 1908 described a child being treated with oral immunotherapy, and a trial of injected peanut showed efficacy in the 1980s. Why has progress been so slow? One reason may relate to the needed focus on safety. The problem with the injection trial was that many people had side effects, including severe anaphylaxis, which essentially halted such research. The earliest studies on oral immunotherapy may have selected people with milder allergies at lower risk for side effects, and some of the trials were not designed properly to draw conclusions. Nonetheless, some people in the early oral immunotherapy studies did not do well. It has become clear that oral immunotherapy studies must be designed with attention to safety and scientific validity, and with long (years) treatment periods, which takes time. Today, studies are highly regulated to ensure the scientific adequacy of the research and the safety of study participants. The delays in investigating the treatments are also due to limited funding and a lack of research volunteers.

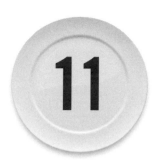

11

How Do I Get **MORE HELP** and **INFORMATION** to Manage Food Allergies?

In this chapter I review how to find key food allergy resources and keep up on food allergy advances and research.

EDUCATIONAL RESOURCES

What should I do to learn more about managing my food allergies?
You made great progress by reading this book. But for additional education, start with your allergist. Make lists of questions to discuss at your next visit. Find out whether other specialists (dietitian, gastroenterologist, counselor, and so on) would be useful to consult. Check the Internet for websites, books, support groups, and organizations.

What types of resources are available for managing life with food allergies?
There are numerous resources. It would take up an entire book just to list them. The following list shows what is out there in a general sense, so you can access or find these resources through the Internet.

How do I know what resources to trust?
Unfortunately, individuals and organizations may provide advice or ser-

Table 11.1
Resources for managing life with food allergies

Resource	Examples
Websites	General about food allergies, specific food allergies (e.g., peanut), professional societies, government agencies, foundations, sites for children, manufacturers catering to food allergy, pharmaceutical companies (emergency medications), blogs, chat rooms.
Books, DVDs, and magazines	Virtually every topic including ones focused on management for children, parents, educators; food-specific (e.g., milk, peanuts, nuts); psychological issues; advice from people living with food allergies; cookbooks; lifestyle magazines.
Apps	Emergency information, management.
Foods	Allergen-free specialty manufacturers; local allergy-friendly restaurants, bakeries; cookbooks, recipes.
Gadgets and practical materials	Carrying cases for medications, allergen labels, examples of allergy-related school forms, medical identification jewelry.
Awareness products	Clothing, stuffed animals, jewelry, wristbands, gifts.

vices that are not necessarily based on good evidence. This is a buyer-beware situation. When it seems too good to be true, it probably is. Consider the source. Is there recognized expertise? Is there external review? For organizations, is there a medical advisory board (there should be), and who are the members? For services, is there a track record? I would suggest special caution in reviewing question-and-answer posts that are not monitored. Sometimes poor or inaccurate advice is dispensed by persons who are not experts in food allergies.

What websites should I use?
The good news about food allergy education and resources is that there has been an explosion of Internet resources. These include major lay and professional organizations, small groups with specific interests in particular food-related illnesses, sites dedicated to specific allergies, preparing

meals, information for restaurants and schools, cooking for persons on restricted diets, and many other topics. There are countless international resources and numerous blogs. It is not feasible to list all the potential resources, but I have included here some key websites that can also form the basis of a gateway to other resources. The list is clearly not exhaustive. I have also included some personal favorites.

Table 11.2
Selected Internet resources on food allergies

Food Allergy Research & Education (FARE)
www.foodallergy.org

A merger of the Food Allergy & Anaphylaxis Network and the Food Allergy Initiative (www.faiusa.org) has resulted in this large lay organization, which partners with many international groups to address all areas of interest in food allergy and anaphylaxis, emphasizing research, education, and advocacy. The website is an excellent gateway to resources.

Consortium of Food Allergy Research
www.cofargroup.org

This is the website of a food allergy research consortium funded by the government. There is a broad selection of downloadable educational materials created by this group.

National Institute of Allergy & Infectious Diseases, Food Allergy Guidelines
www.niaid.nih.gov/topics/foodallergy

From this page, you can access materials created by or in concert with the Expert Panel's *Guidelines for the Diagnosis and Management of Food Allergies in the U.S.*

The FDA and Its Center for Food Safety and Applied Nutrition
www.fda.gov/Food
www.fda.gov/aboutfda/centersoffices/officeoffoods/cfsan/default.htm

The FDA provides a comprehensive listing of useful information about government-related notifications on food safety and allergen issues.

Centers for Disease Control: Food Allergies in Schools
www.cdc.gov/HealthyYouth/foodallergies

Learn more about CDC educational materials and initiatives related to food allergies in schools.

Selected Internet resources on food allergies

FPIES Foundation
www.thefpiesfoundation.org

The International Association for Food Protein Enterocolitis
www.iaffpe.org

These are the websites of two lay organizations focused on food protein-induced enterocolitis syndrome.

American Partnership for Eosinophilic Disorders
http://apfed.org

This lay organization focuses on eosinophilic disorders, such as eosinophilic esophagitis.

Kids with Food Allergies Foundation
www.kidswithfoodallergies.org

Families of children with food allergies can find support and an online forum on this website.

National Eczema Association
www.nationaleczema.org

Inflammatory Skin Disease Institute
www.isdionline.org

Coalition of Skin Diseases
www.coalitionofskindiseases.org

These lay organizations focusing on allergic skin diseases provide multiple resources for information and support.

Asthma and Allergy Network, Mothers of Asthmatics
www.aanma.org

Focusing on asthma and allergies, this lay organization offers resources and support.

Jaffe Food Allergy Institute at Mount Sinai
www.mssm.edu/research/programs/jaffe-food-allergy-institute

At the author's institutional homepage, you will find updates on research and clinical care.

Clinical Trials.gov
www.clinicaltrials.gov

Learn about ongoing research studies and how you can participate in food allergy research. Search according to your interests, such as "food allergy" or "peanut allergy."

continued

Table 11.2 *continued*
Selected Internet resources on food allergies

American Academy of Allergy, Asthma, and Immunology
www.aaaai.org

A professional medical organization, the AAAAI provides resources for the public as well.

American College of Allergy, Asthma, and Immunology
www.acaai.org

This site is home of another professional medical organization with resources for the public.

Asthma and Allergy Foundation of America
www.aafa.org

This website is hosted by a lay organization focusing on allergic diseases and asthma.

American Academy of Pediatrics
www.aap.org

This well-known professional medical organization has extensive pediatric resources.

American Dietetic Association
www.eatright.org

Here you'll find information on nutritional issues from a professional organization of dietitians.

MedicAlert
www.medicalert.org

MedicAlert is a standard resource for obtaining medical identification jewelry.

Anaphylaxis Canada
www.anaphylaxis.ca

Anaphylaxis Campaign (UK)
www.anaphylaxis.org.uk

EuroPrevall
www.europrevall.org

Worldwide, there are numerous lay and professional organizations focusing on food allergy and anaphylaxis.

Is there an app for food allergy?

There are many, and the list of types continues to grow. You can find apps that scan bar codes and relay food allergen information, present information about related foods, track symptoms and diet, and provide interactive recipes. I encourage you to explore the increasing variety of apps for food allergy, but use caution. Some are not based on medical evidence regarding food allergies. For example, botanically related foods are not necessarily all off limits to a person allergic to one from a related group, as one app claims. Some apps provide restaurant food ingredients, but I urge caution. Discuss each meal separately with staff and do not rely solely on an app. Some of the apps are based on notions of symptom relationships to foods that are unproven (for example some behavioral aspects, fatigue, and so forth). Keeping apps up to date is also an issue, so it is important to double-check ingredient labels when following advice on shopping from an app.

What should I do to educate my allergic child about food allergies?

Again, start with your allergist for specific information. It is okay to ask your allergist, "Can you explain more about the allergy to my child?" There are books, websites, and programs specifically aimed toward children. A good place to begin is at www.foodallergy.org. They have links to programs, newsletters, activities, and books for children and teenagers.

What can I do to educate my family about food allergies?

Sharing resources that you found to be helpful is a great start. Bring interested relatives to an allergist visit as well. There are books designed to introduce siblings and relatives to the basics of food allergy.

What should I do to educate others about food allergies?

Usually, a health care provider at a school or camp will be responsible for staff education. If there has not already been progress, however, you may wish to make that person aware of educational programs. New online programs with interactive educational features for teachers and others are available. Check the website, www.foodallergy.org.

How can I educate schools or camps about food allergies?

You may wish to point them to educational materials mentioned above and in chapter 6. A nice source of interactive learning is www.allergy ready.com, which has interactive educational materials for free. How to C.A.R.E. for Students with Food Allergies online Anaphylaxis Readiness Course has been developed in partnership with leading food allergy organizations and health care professionals to improve the quality of school personnel education. I reviewed this excellent program as well.

SUPPORT GROUPS, ADVOCACY, AND RESEARCH

What organizations provide laypersons with information about research, advocacy, and support?

There are many, but leading the charge in the United States have been the Food Allergy & Anaphylaxis Network, with twenty years of dedicated work, and the Food Allergy Initiative, with over a decade of experience. To better focus efforts on research, advocacy, and education, these two organizations have recently merged into one large one called Food Allergy Research & Education (FARE).

Are there support groups for food allergies?

Yes, and you can search for them using the "Support Group Lookup Tool" at www.foodallergy.org.

How would I start a support group on food allergies?

You might start by talking to your allergist and others in your community who are interested. FARE is another resource.

How can I learn about advocacy for food allergies?

Check www.foodallergy.org. Advocacy activities, led in part by lay organizations, have achieved improved allergen food labeling, increased government research grants, improved school programs, better access to epinephrine in an emergency, and more effective approaches to food allergies in restaurants. But there is still much to do, and you can help.

How can I learn about participating in research studies about food allergies?
Check out Food Allergy Research & Education and ClinicalTrials.gov, as listed previously.

HANDY FORMS

What types of form letters or plans should I obtain from my doctor?
The two most common forms are the emergency action plan and a travel letter. Versions are available from www.foodallergy.org. Examples are shown here.

Figure 11.1
Travel Letter

DATE

RE: [Name, Date of Birth]

To Whom It May Concern:
My Patient named above suffers from life-threatening food allergies. This is a severe allergy that makes it medically necessary to carry an antihistamine and self-injectable epinephrine. Epinephrine is prescribed by a licensed medical professional and my patient needs to have this life-saving medication available at all times, Including during travel. A food allergic reaction can result in severe symptoms and this medication is needed promptly. Please allow my patient to have the self-injectable epinephrine and additional medications (antihistamine and asthma medications, if needed) on board the airplane. Because of the food allergies, my patient may need to carry sufficient food as well.

Sincerely,

_____   _____, M.D.

Figure 11.2
Food Allergy Action Plan

Food Allergy Action Plan
Emergency Care Plan

Place
Student's
Picture
Here

Name: _____ D.O.B.: ___ / ___ / ___

Allergy to: _____

Weight: _____ lbs.   **Asthma:** ☐ Yes (higher risk for a severe reaction) ☐ No

Extremely reactive to the following foods: _____
THEREFORE:
☐ If checked, give epinephrine immediately for ANY symptoms if the allergen was *likely* eaten.
☐ If checked, give epinephrine immediately if the allergen was *definitely* eaten, even if no symptoms are noted.

Any SEVERE SYMPTOMS after suspected or known ingestion:

One or more of the following:
LUNG: Short of breath, wheeze, repetitive cough
HEART: Pale, blue, faint, weak pulse, dizzy, confused
THROAT: Tight, hoarse, trouble breathing/swallowing
MOUTH: Obstructive swelling (tongue and/or lips)
SKIN: Many hives over body

Or **combination** of symptoms from different body areas:
SKIN: Hives, itchy rashes, swelling (e.g., eyes, lips)
GUT: Vomiting, diarrhea, crampy pain

1. **INJECT EPINEPHRINE IMMEDIATELY**
2. Call 911
3. Begin monitoring (see box below)
4. Give additional medications:*
    -Antihistamine
    -Inhaler (bronchodilator) if asthma

*Antihistamines & inhalers/bronchodilators are not to be depended upon to treat a severe reaction (anaphylaxis). USE EPINEPHRINE.

MILD SYMPTOMS ONLY:

MOUTH: Itchy mouth
SKIN: A few hives around mouth/face, mild itch
GUT: Mild nausea/discomfort

1. **GIVE ANTIHISTAMINE**
2. Stay with student; alert healthcare professionals and parent
3. If symptoms progress (see above), USE EPINEPHRINE
4. Begin monitoring (see box below)

Medications/Doses
Epinephrine (brand and dose): _____
Antihistamine (brand and dose): _____
Other (e.g., inhaler-bronchodilator if asthmatic): _____

Monitoring
Stay with student; alert healthcare professionals and parent. Tell rescue squad epinephrine was given; request an ambulance with epinephrine. Note time when epinephrine was administered. A second dose of epinephrine can be given 5 minutes or more after the first if symptoms persist or recur. For a severe reaction, consider keeping student lying on back with legs raised. Treat student even if parents cannot be reached. See back/attached for auto-injection technique.

_____   _____   _____   _____
Parent/Guardian Signature   Date   Physician/Healthcare Provider Signature   Date

TURN FORM OVER   Form provided courtesy of the Food Allergy & Anaphylaxis Network (www.foodallergy.org) 9/2011

Food Allergy Action Plan (page 2)

EPIPEN Auto-Injector and EPIPEN Jr Auto-Injector Directions

- First, remove the EPIPEN Auto-Injector from the plastic carrying case
- Pull off the blue safety release cap

- Hold orange tip near outer thigh (always apply to thigh)

- Swing and firmly push orange tip against outer thigh. Hold on thigh for approximately 10 seconds. Remove the EPIPEN Auto-Injector and massage the area for 10 more seconds

EPIPEN 2·PAK® EPIPEN Jr 2·PAK®
(Epinephrine) Auto-Injectors 0.3/0.15mg

DEY® and the Dey logo, EpiPen®, EpiPen 2-Pak®, and EpiPen Jr 2-Pak® are registered trademarks of Dey Pharma, L.P.

Adrenaclick™ 0.3 mg and Adrenaclick™ 0.15 mg Directions

Remove GREY caps labeled "1" and "2."

Place RED rounded tip against outer thigh, press down hard until needle penetrates. Hold for 10 seconds, then remove

A food allergy response kit should contain at least two doses of epinephrine, other medications as noted by the student's physician, and a copy of this Food Allergy Action Plan.

A kit must accompany the student if he/she is off school grounds (i.e., field trip).

Contacts

Call 911 (Rescue squad: (___) _____-_____) Doctor: _____   Phone: (___) _____-_____
Parent/Guardian: _____   Phone: (___) _____-_____

Other Emergency Contacts
Name/Relationship: _____   Phone: (___) _____-_____
Name/Relationship: _____   Phone: (___) _____-_____

Form provided courtesy of the Food Allergy & Anaphylaxis Network (www.foodallergy.org) 9/2011

SELECTED MEDICAL REFERENCES

Boyce JA, Assa'ad A, Burks AW, Jones SM, Sampson HA, Wood RA et al. Guidelines for the diagnosis and management of food allergy in the United States: report of the NIAID-sponsored expert panel. J Allergy Clin Immunol 2010; 126(6 Suppl):S1–58.

Greer FR, Sicherer SH, Burks AW. Effects of early nutritional interventions on the development of atopic disease in infants and children: the role of maternal dietary restriction, breast-feeding, timing of introduction of complementary foods, and hydrolyzed formulas. Pediatrics 2008; 121(1):183–91.

Liacouras CA, Furuta GT, Hirano I, Atkins D, Attwood SE, Bonis PA et al. Eosinophilic esophagitis: updated consensus recommendations for children and adults. J Allergy Clin Immunol 2011; 128(1):3–20.

Lieberman JA, Weiss C, Furlong TJ, Sicherer M, Sicherer SH. Bullying among pediatric patients with food allergy. Ann Allergy Asthma Immunol 2010; 105(4):282–6.

Nowak-Wegrzyn A, Assa'ad AH, Bahna SL, Bock SA, Sicherer SH, Teuber SS. Work Group report: oral food challenge testing. J Allergy Clin Immunol 2009; 123(6 Suppl):S365–S383.

Sampson MA, Muñoz-Furlong A, Sicherer SH. Risk-taking and coping strategies of adolescents and young adults with food allergy. J Allergy Clin Immunol 2006; 117(6):1440–5.

Sicherer SH. Epidemiology of food allergy. J Allergy Clin Immunol 2011; 127(3):594–602.

Sicherer SH. Food protein–induced enterocolitis syndrome: case presentations and management lessons. J Allergy Clin Immunol 2005; 115(1):149–56.

Sicherer SH, Muñoz-Furlong A, Godbold JH, Sampson HA. U.S. prevalence of self-reported peanut, tree nut, and sesame allergy: 11-year follow-up. J Allergy Clin Immunol 2010; 125(6):1322–6.

Sicherer SH, Sampson HA. Food allergy. J Allergy Clin Immunol 2010; 125(2 Suppl 2):S116–S125.

Sicherer SH, Sampson HA. Food allergy: recent advances in pathophysiology and treatment. Annu Rev Med 2009; 60:261–77.

Sicherer SH, Simons FE. Self-injectable epinephrine for first-aid management of anaphylaxis. Pediatrics 2007; 119(3):638–46.

Sicherer SH, Vargas PA, Groetch ME, Christie L, Carlisle SK, Noone S, Jones SM. Development and validation of educational materials for food allergy. J Pediatr 2012;160(4):651–6.

Sicherer SH, Wood RA. Allergy testing in childhood: Using allergen specific tests. Pediatrics 2012; 129(1):193–7.

Young MC, Muñoz-Furlong A, Sicherer SH. Management of food allergies in schools: a perspective for allergists. J Allergy Clin Immunol 2009; 124(2):175–82, 182.

INDEX

acid blocking medication, 146

action plans. *See* emergency plans

additives, 43–44

adverse reactions, reporting, 164

advisory statements, 162–63

advocacy activities, 266–67

affinity testing, 89–90

age: anaphylaxis and, 95, 98–100; blood tests and, 70; food allergy management and, 189–91

airborne food proteins, 153, 222

airplane travel, 187–88

ALCAT tests, 88

alcoholic beverages, 41–42

"allergic march," 236

allergic reactions, avoiding: age-related tasks for, 189–91; amounts that trigger reactions, 152; at camp, 184–85; from casual exposure, 153–57; from cross-contact, 151–52; at home, 157–59; from manufactured products, 159–64; overview of, 149–50; peanut-sniffing dogs, 195–96; from relationships, 188–89; at restaurants, 164–68; at school, 169–84; at social events, 168–69; special exposure risks, 192–94; when traveling, 186–88; at work, 185–86

allergists, 50, 54–55

alternative therapies, 56–57

American Academy of Allergy, Asthma, and Immunology, 54, 264

American Board of Allergy and Immunology, 55

American College of Allergy, Asthma, and Immunology, 54, 264

anaphylaxis: antihistamines for, 108–10; asthma and, 92, 94, 96, 98, 115; course of allergies causing, 217; described, 4, 91, 101; fatal, risks for, 95–96; food-associated exercise-induced, 7, 98, 118, 217; foods causing, 91; illnesses mimicking, 94, oral food challenges and, 80; predicting, 115–16; preparating for, 97–98, 113–15; risks for, 98–100; skin tests to foods causing, 64; symptoms of, 92–93, 94–95; treating, 97, 111–13, 116–17, 118–19, 251; triggers for, 93. *See also* epinephrine

anisakis allergy, 38

antifungal therapy, 253–54

antihistamines: described, 108; effects of, 109, 110; side effects of, 109; skin tests and, 64–65; types of, 108

anti-IgE therapy, 243–44

anxiety: hyperventilation and, 200–201; reducing risk of, 202–3; resistance to eating caused by, 201–2; severity of, 199–200; symptoms of, 213; touch tests for, 200; treating, 203; in young children, 203–4

applied kinesiology tests, 86

apps for food allergy, 265

arthritis, 148

aspartame, 45

asthma: anaphylaxis and, 92, 94, 96, 98, 115; food allergy and, 121; medications for, 111

auriculotemporal syndrome, 12

autism, 147

autoinjectors of epinephrine, 103–4, 105–7

avoiding allergic reactions. *See* allergic reactions, avoiding

baking foods, 19, 21, 249

Barrett, Stephen, 58

basophil activation tests, 85

beans, 13, 32–33. *See also* peanuts; soy allergy
behavior and food, 9, 148
benzoates, 45
BHA/BHT, 45
biopsies, 143
blood tests: accuracy of, 70; age and, 70; described, 67–68; food allergy panel, 71–72; number of foods tested, 71; for resolution of allergy, 218; results of, 68–70, 74; severity of allergy and, 73; skin tests compared to, 70–71, 73
blood transfusions, 194
Bock, Allan, xvii
breast feeding, 192–93, 229–32
bronchodilators, 111
bullying, 205–7
bus transport and schools, 177–78

cafeterias in schools, 175, 176–77
calcium intake, 210
calorie intake, inadequate, 207–8
camp, avoiding allergic reactions at, 184–85
carbohydrate intake, 209
celiac disease, 24, 132–33
cell phones, ICE (In Case of Emergency) on, 115
charcoal, activated, for anaphylaxis, 113
chef cards for restaurant dining, 165
Chinese herbal remedies, 244, 258
chitosan, 40
chocolate, 23
chronic illnesses: atopic dermatitis, 6, 84, 124–27, 217; celiac disease, 24, 132–33; colic, constipation, irritable bowel syndrome, and reflux, 128–32; enterocolitis, 7, 84, 135–41, 251; eosinophilic esophagitis, 7, 84, 142–46, 217, 251; food protein enteropathy and protein intolerance, 141; gastrointestinal or digestive, 127–28; hives, 121–24; not related to food allergies, 147–48; overview of, 120; proctocolitis, 133–35; respiratory symptoms, 121
clinical trials, 240, 242, 254–57
cocoa, 23
coconut, 26
colic, 128–30
college, allergy management at, 183–84
colors, synthetic, 44
component testing, 86, 88–89
constipation, 130
"contains" statements on labels, 161
cooking foods, 16, 159, 249
corticosteroids for anaphylaxis, 111–12
cow's milk, 20–23, 214, 215
cross-contact, 151–52
cytotoxic testing, 88

dating relationships, 188–89
delayed allergic reactions, 147, 226–27
Department of Agriculture website, 210
depression, 202, 203
dermatitis, atopic, 6, 84, 124–27, 217
development of new food allergies, 219–20, 236–37
diagnosis, tests in, 59–60, 67
diet: during breast feeding, 230; elemental diets, 76–77; nutrition and, 207–12; during pregnancy, 228–29; for prevention, 226, 233–35; rotation diets, 252. *See also* elimination diets
dietitians, 55, 212
diet records, 51
digestive illnesses, 127–28
diseases. *See* chronic illnesses; illnesses
dishes, cleaning, 158
doctors: deciding when to talk to, 49–50; finding, 54–55; preparing for visits to, 50–54
dogs, peanut-sniffing, 195–96
double-blind, placebo-controlled oral food challenge, xvii–xviii, 81

eating, fear of, 201–2, 207

eczema, allergic, 6, 124–27, 217
educational resources, 260–66
eggs, 18–20, 154, 214, 215–16
elemental diets, 76–77
elimination diets: described, 74; for
  eosinophilic esophagitis, 145;
  example of, 76; illnesses tested,
  74–75; immune system-boosting,
  254; nutrition and, 208; risks of, 75
emergency plans: for anaphylaxis,
  97–98, 113–15; form for, 268–69;
  for schools, 179–80
emergency room treatment for
  anaphylaxis, 97
emotional concerns, 199–204
enterocolitis, 7, 84, 135–41, 251
enteropathy, 7, 132–33, 141
environmental influences, 225–26
eosinophilic gut disease, 7, 142. *See also*
  esophagitis, eosinophilic
eosinophils, 142
epicutaneous immunotherapy, 249–50
epilepsy, 147
epinephrine: accidental finger injection
  of, 107–8; administering, 102,
  180–82; autoinjectors of, 103–4,
  105–7; delayed treatment with, 95, 99;
  doses of, 103, 104, 106–7; effectiveness of, 104; effects of, 103; fear of
  self-injection, 107; injections of,
  101–2, 116–17; interactions with, 105;
  for PFIES, 137; prescriptions for, 101;
  on school buses, 178; side effects of,
  104–5; storing, 106, 180, visit to ER
  after injection of, 97
epitope testing, 89
esophagitis, eosinophilic, 7, 84, 142–46,
  217, 251
exercise, food, and anaphylaxis, 7, 98,
  118, 217
exposure, noningestion, 222

FAAN (Food Allergy & Anaphylaxis
  Network), xviii, 100

FAEIA (food-associated exercise-
  induced anaphylaxis), 7, 98, 118
FALCPA (Food Allergen Labeling and
  Consumer Protection Act, 2004),
  160, 161
family gatherings, avoiding allergic
  reactions during, 168–69
family relationships, effects on, 204
FARE (Food Allergy Research and
  Education), xv, 262, 266, 272
fat intake, 209, 235
fear: of eating, 201–2, 207; of self-
  injection, 107
Federal Food, Drug, and Cosmetic Act,
  160
feeding tests. *See* oral food challenges
field trips, 178
fish, 11, 36–38, 155–56, 214, 216
504 plans, 182–83
flour, substitute, 24
Food Allergen Labeling and Consumer
  Protection Act (FALCPA, 2004), 160,
  161
food allergies: causes and triggers of, 3,
  15–17, 152; defined, 1; development
  of new, 219–20, 236–37; evolution in
  understanding of, xvii–xviii; immune
  system in, 1–2, 221, 223–24; increase
  in, xviii, 14; information on, xviii–xix;
  prevalence of, 14; recurrence of, 219.
  See also avoiding allergic reactions;
  prevention; resolution of food
  allergies; severity of food allergy;
  symptoms; treatment
Food Allergy & Anaphylaxis Network
  (FAAN), xviii, 100
Food Allergy Initiative, xviii, 258
Foodallergy.org website, 165
Food Allergy Research and Education
  (FARE), xv, 262, 266, 272
Food and Drug Administration (FDA)
  website, 163, 164, 262
food intolerance, 2
food poisoning, 2

food protein enteropathy, 7, 141
food protein-induced enterocolitis (FPIES), 135–41, 217, 251
food protein-induced proctocolitis, 133–35
food protein intolerance, 141
foods: baking, 19, 21, 249; cooking, 16, 159, 249; suspect, taking to doctor visits, 53. *See also* oral food challenges; *specific foods*
formulas for babies, 23, 230–32
FPIES (food protein-induced enterocolitis), 135–41, 217, 251
"free from" statements on labels, 161
fructose, 13–14
fruits, 34, 216

gastritis, eosinophilic, 142
gastroenteritis, eosinophilic, 142
gastroesophageal reflux disease (GERD), 131–32
gastrointestinal illnesses, 127–28
gelatin, 38, 42–43
genetic influences, 224–26
gluten-sensitive enteropathy, 132–33
grain allergy, 24–25. *See also* wheat allergy
grocery shopping, 157. *See also* labels

hair analysis, 87
hand washing, 174
hay fever, 121
headaches, 9–10, 147–48
help, seeking, 46
herbal treatments, 57, 244, 258
histamine skin tests, 61
hives, 7, 93, 96, 121–24, 156
home, avoiding allergic reactions in, 157–59
honey, 42
hospital meals, 194
hygiene hypothesis, 224, 236, 238, 245
hyperventilation, 10, 119, 200–201

IBS (irritable bowel syndrome), 130–31
ICE (In Case of Emergency) on cell phones, 115
IgE antibodies, 1–2, 62, 85
IgG/IgG4 testing, 87
IHCP (individualized health care plan), 183
illnesses: attributed wrongly to allergies, 9–14; overview of, 4, 217. *See also* chronic illnesses; symptoms; *specific illnesses*
immune system, 1–2, 221, 223–24
immunotherapy: epicutaneous, 249–50; injections, 246; oral and sublingual, 247–49, 259; for pollen allergy, 237
individualized health care plan (IHCP), 183
infants: autoinjectors for, 107; breast feeding, 192–93, 229–32; colic in, 128–30; enterocolitis in, 135–41; exposure of to whole proteins, 226; formulas for, 23, 230–32; procto-colitis in, 133–35; solid food intro-duction, 232
ingredient information, obtaining, 52, 163, 165
intercourse, 189
Internet resources, 262–64
interpersonal relationships: dating, 188–89; family, 168–69, 204; peer, 205–7; spousal, 204–5
intradermal tests, 85
iodide, 16, 39
irritable bowel syndrome (IBS), 130–31

Jaffe Food Allergy Institute, xviii, 263
jewelry, medical identification, 114, 171

kissing, 188–89
kIU/L, 68

labels on food products, 159–64
lactose intolerance, 2, 12–13
laser therapy, 253

latex, 47
LEAP (Learning Early About Peanut allergy) study, 237
legumes, 32–33. *See also* peanuts
Li, Xiu-Min, 244, 258
lifestyle: effects on, 197; hygiene hypothesis and, 224, 236, 238, 245; nutrition, 207–12. *See also* quality of life
lupine/lupin, 17, 32
lychee/lichee, 26

mammalian meat allergy, 35–36
May, Charles, xvii
meats, 35–36, 157, 216
MedicAlert website, 114, 264
medical history, 53–54, 59–60
medical identification jewelry, 114, 171, 264
medical issues. *See* illnesses; medications; symptoms
medical references, 270–71
medications: acid blocking, 146; discontinuing before doctor visits, 52–53; with egg, 20; for eosinophilic esophagitis, 145; food allergens in, 193; with lactose, 22–23; at schools, 180–82; skin tests and, 64–65; with soy lecithin, 32; steroids, 111–12, 145; taking to doctor visits, 53. *See also* antihistamines; epinephrine
mental health concerns, 201–4. *See also* anxiety
mercury amalgam removal, 253
milk from cows, 20–23, 214, 215
montelukast (Singulair), 112
MSG (monosodium glutamate), 44–45
Muñoz-Furlong, Anne, xviii

natural remedies, 57. *See also* herbal treatments
nickel, 48
nitrates, 45
nutrition, 207–12. *See also* diet

nutritionists, 56. *See also* registered dietitians
nuts, 6, 151. *See also* peanuts; tree nuts

occupation and food allergies, 7–8
oral allergy syndrome, 4–6, 217, 222, 251
oral food challenges: described, 77; double-blind, placebo-controlled, xvii–xviii, 81; emotional consequences of, 84; number of foods tested, 79; preparing for, 81–82; reactions to, 82–83; in research, 256–57; results from, 83–84; symptoms and reactions to, 79–81; uses of, 77–79
orthomolecular therapy, 252–53

parabens, 45
paraprofessionals in schools, 177
parasites, 245
patch tests, 84–85
peanuts: allergy to, 16, 17–18, 214, 215; differences in allergy rates, 238; fatal food anaphylaxis and, 96; skin exposure to, 234; soy allergy and, 30–31
peanut-sniffing dogs, 195–96
pectin, 44
peer relationships and bullying, 205–7
phytoestrogens, 212
platelet-activating factor, 116
pollen-associated food (oral) allergy syndrome, 4–6, 217, 222, 251
poultry allergy, 35
prebiotics, 244–45
pregnancy diets, 228–29
preservatives, 43, 45
prevention: breast feeding and formulas, 229–32; delay compared to, 227; dietary recommendations for, 226, 233–35; environment issues and, 225–26; genetic issues and, 224–26; nondietary recommendations for,

prevention *(continued)*
235–37; overview of, 223–24;
pregnancy diets, 228–29; solid food
introduction, 232; strategies for,
227–28; studies of, 237; worldwide
observations on, 238
probiotics, 236, 238, 244–45
proctocolitis, 7, 133–35
product labels, 159–64
protein intake, 208–9
provocation-neutralization tests,
86–87, 252
pseudoallergens, 122–23
psoralens, 11
pulse tests, 88

Quackwatch website, 58
quality of life: emotional concerns,
199–204; health-related, 197–98;
impact on, 198–99; improving, 198,
213; interpersonal relationships,
204–7; nutrition, 207–12
questions for doctors, 51

radiocontrast dyes, 39
recurrence of food allergies, 219
reflux, 131–32, 146
registered dietitians, 55, 212
research: Chinese herbal remedies, 244,
258; overview of, 239–43; participation in, 254–57, 267; prevention,
challenges of, 237; progress of, 259;
on vaccines for food allergies, 246
resistance testing, 87
resolution of food allergies: causes of,
221; evaluations for, 218; factors
affecting, 220–21; illnesses caused by,
217; overview of, 214; predicting, 215;
recurrence or development of new
allergies after, 219–20
resources: educational, 260–66; forms,
267–69; medical references, 270–71;
support groups, advocacy, and
research, 266–67

respiratory symptoms, 121. *See also*
asthma; hyperventilation
restaurants, avoiding allergic reactions
at, 164–68
rotation diets, 252

salt water skin tests, 62
scarring from eosinophilic esophagitis,
146
schools: approaching about allergies,
169–70, 171; banning allergens at,
174; bullying in, 205–7; bus transportation and, 177–78; cafeterias in, 175,
176–77; cleaning of, 175; emergency
management plans in, 179–80; field
trips from, 178; 504 plans, 182–83;
guidelines for allergy management in,
170–71; handwashing in, 174;
paraprofessionals in, 177; resources
for, 266; responsibility for allergy
management of, 172–73; snack times
in, 175–76; student responsibility for
allergy management, 173–74
scombroid fish poisoning, 11, 37
Section 504 plans, 182–83
seeds, 29–30
self-injection, 107, 180–82
sesame allergy, 29–30, 74
severity of food allergy: blood tests and,
73; overview of, 8; predicting, 115–16;
resolution and, 220; skin tests and, 67
sexual relationships, 189
shellfish, 38–40, 155–57, 214, 216
Sicherer, Mati, 205–7
Singulair (montelukast), 112
skin exposure, 234
skin tests: accuracy of, 62, 65, 66, 70;
blood tests compared to, 70–71, 73;
described, 60–61; foods used for, 61;
histamine, 61; number of, 65–66;
procedure for, 62–63; for resolution
of allergies, 218; response to, 63, 67;
results of, 66; risks from, 63–64;
salt water, 62

smell and allergic reactions, 153, 154, 195

snack times in schools, 175–76

social outings, avoiding allergic reactions during, 168–69

sorbates, 45

soy allergy, 30–32, 214, 216

soy drinks, 212

spices, 40–41

spousal relationships, effects on, 204–5

starches, 33–34

steroids, 111–12, 145

storing epinephrine, 106, 180

sulfites, 45–46

support groups, 266

swelling, 47

swimming pools, 156

symptoms: of anxiety, 213; evaluating, 50; oral food challenges and, 79–81; overview of, 3–8; recording, 50; talking to doctors about, 49; unusual reactions, 47–48; wrongly attributed to allergies, 9–14. *See also* anaphylaxis; hives; hyperventilation

synbiotics, 244–45

tartrazine, 44

taste tests, 150

teenagers and risk for anaphylaxis, 98–100

tests: affinity, 89–90; basophil activation, 85; biopsies, 143; component, 85, 88–89; elimination diets, 74–77; epitope, 89; for evaluation, 54; intradermal, 85; oral food challenges, 77–84; overview of, 59–60; patch, 84–85; provocation-neutralization, 86–87, 252; total IgE, 85; touch, 200; unexpected results from, 90;

unproven and disproven, 58, 86–88. *See also* blood tests; skin tests

touch and allergic reactions, 153–54, 195

translational research, 242

travel, 186–88, 267

treatment: general approaches to, 243–45; herbal, 57, 244, 258; of illnesses, 251; immunotherapy, 237, 259; natural, 57; specific approaches to, 246–50; unproven, 251–54

tree nuts: acorns and, 155; allergy to, 25–29, 214; course of allergy to, 215; fatal food anaphylaxis and, 96; peanut allergy and, 18

triggers of food allergy, 3, 15–17, 152

TSO (*Trichuris suis ova*), 245

Understanding and Managing Your Child's Food Allergies (Sicherer), xiii

unusual reactions to food, 47–48

urine autoinjection, 253

urticaria, 7, 121–24, 156. *See also* hives

U.S. Department of Agriculture website, 210

U.S. Food and Drug Administration (FDA) website, 163, 164, 262

vaccines: with egg, 20; food allergens in, 193–94; for food allergies, 246

VEGA testing, 87

vegetables, 33–34, 216

vitamin D, 209–10, 235

water, drinking, 156–57

weight loss, 207–8

wheat allergy, 24–25, 214, 216

work, avoiding allergic reactions at, 185–86

ABOUT THE AUTHOR

Scott H. Sicherer, M.D., is a professor of pediatrics at the Mount Sinai School of Medicine and a researcher in the Jaffe Food Allergy Institute at Mount Sinai. He is Chief of the Division of Pediatric Allergy and Immunology. Dr. Sicherer received his medical degree with honors from the Johns Hopkins University School of Medicine and his pediatric training, including a chief residency, at Mount Sinai in New York City. He completed a fellowship in allergy and immunology at Johns Hopkins and then returned as faculty to Mount Sinai. He is board-certified in pediatrics and in allergy and immunology and specializes in food allergies. His research interests, funded by the National Institutes of Health, Food Allergy Initiative, and the Food Allergy & Anaphylaxis Network, include allergic diseases caused by specific foods, such as peanuts, tree nuts, eggs, seafood, and milk; the natural history of food allergy; atopic dermatitis; gastrointestinal manifestations of food allergies; epidemiology of food allergy; psychosocial issues associated with food allergies; modalities to educate physicians and parents about food allergy; and the genetics of food allergy. He has published over 130 articles in scientific journals and has authored numerous book chapters in major pediatric and allergy textbooks. He is a medical advisor to Food Allergy Research & Education (FARE) and others. He is past chair of the Adverse Reactions to Foods Committee of the Academy of Allergy, Asthma, and Immunology and past chair of the Section on Allergy and Immunology of the American Academy of Pediatrics. He is associate editor of the *Journal of Allergy and Clinical Immunology* and of its sister journal, *JACI: In Practice*, and is on the board of directors of the American Board of Allergy and Immunology. He has authored a children's book on food allergy, *Maya and Andrew Learn About Food Allergies*; co-authored a book about peanut allergy, *The Complete Peanut Allergy Handbook*, and another about milk allergy, *The Complete Idiot's Guide to Dairy Free Eating*; and written a comprehensive book about food allergy for parents, *Understanding and Managing Your Child's Food Allergies*. Dr. Sicherer has been consistently recognized as a "Top Doctor" by Castle-Connolly/*New York Magazine*, and been recognized by *U.S. News and World Report* as being among the top 1% of pediatric allergists. He lectures extensively on food allergy topics to various professional and lay organizations and has had numerous television and radio appearances to discuss food allergy.

He participates as a guest providing "Ask the Expert" answers for *Allergic Living* magazine, Sharecare.com, Food Allergy Research & Education (www.foodallergy.org), and the American Academy of Allergy, Asthma, and Immunology.